Council on Chiropractic Practice

Clinical Practice Guideline

Number 1

Vertebral Subluxation in Chiropractic Practice

1998

Clinical Practice Guideline:
Vertebral Subluxation
in Chiropractic Practice

Published by:
Council on Chiropractic Practice

Library of Congress Catalog Number: 98-073514
ISBN: 0-9666598-0-5

Panel Members

Christopher Kent, D.C., F.C.C.I.
President, Council on
  Chiropractic Practice
Post-graduate Faculty
Life University, Marietta, Georgia
Ramsey, New Jersey

William Ralph Boone, Ph.D., D.C.
Vice President, Council on
  Chiropractic Practice
Editor, Journal of Vertebral
  Subluxation Research
Irvine, California

Terry A. Rondberg, D.C.
Secretary, Council on
  Chiropractic Practice
President, World Chiropractic Alliance
Chandler, Arizona

Harold G. McCoy, D.C.
Treasurer, Council on
  Chiropractic Practice
President, International
  Spinal Health Institute
Private Practice
Kirkland, Washington

Emmanuel T. Akporiaye, Ph.D.
Associate Professor of Microbiology
  and Immunology
Arizona Health Sciences Center
University of Arizona
Tucson, Arizona

Robert Blanks, Ph.D.
Professor, Department of Anatomy and
  Neurobiology
University of California, Irvine
Irvine, California

Patrick Gentempo, D.C.
President, Chiropractic
  Leadership Alliance
Paterson, New Jersey

John J. Gerhardt, M.D.
Consultant in Physical Medicine
  and Rehabilitation
Shriners Hospital and Veterans Affairs
Hospital Medical Center
Portland, Oregon

Veronica Gutierrez, D.C.
Member of the Washington State
  Quality Assurance Commission
Private Practice
Arlington, Washington

Jonathan Hatch, Esquire
Member Washington State
  Bar Association
Member Snohomish County
  Bar Association
Lynnwood, Washington

Jay Holder, D.C., M.D., Ph.D.
President, American College of
Addictionology and Compulsive
  Disorders
Private Practice
Miami Beach, Florida

Carol James
Consumer Member
Bellevue, Washington

Matthew McCoy, D.C.
Vice President,
  International Spinal Health Institute
Private Practice
Kirkland, Washington

Stephen F. Renner, D.C.
Member American Board of
  Forensic Examiners
Private Practice
Spokane, Washington

Steven Shochat, D.C.
Private Practice
Tucson, Arizona

Contents

Introduction and Methodology

The Council on Chiropractic Practice

In the summer of 1995, chiropractic history was made in Phoenix, Arizona with the formation of the Council on Chiropractic Practice (CCP). The meeting was attended by an interdisciplinary assembly of distinguished chiropractors, medical physicians, basic scientists, attorneys, and consumer representatives.

The CCP is an apolitical, non-profit organization. It is not affiliated with any other chiropractic association. The CCP represents a grass-roots movement to produce practice guidelines which serve the needs of the consumer, and are consistent with "real world" chiropractic practice.

The mission of the CCP is "To develop evidence-based guidelines, conduct research and perform other functions that will enhance the practice of chiropractic for the benefit of the consumer."

Evidence-Based Practice

Evidence-based clinical practice is defined as "The conscientious, explicit, and judicious use of the current best evidence in making decisions about the care of individual patients... (it) is not restricted to randomized trials and meta-analyses. It involves tracking down the best external evidence with which to answer our clinical questions." [1]

This concept was embraced by the Association of Chiropractic Colleges in its first position paper. This paper stated:

> Chiropractic is concerned with the preservation and restoration of health, and focuses particular attention on the subluxation.
>
> A subluxation is a complex of functional and/or structural and/or pathological articular changes that compromise neural integrity and may influence organ system function and general health.
>
> A subluxation is evaluated, diagnosed, and managed through the use of chiropractic procedures based on the best available rational and empirical evidence. [2]

The CCP has developed practice guidelines for vertebral subluxation with the active participation of field doctors, consultants, seminar leaders, and technique experts. In addition, the Council has utilized the services of interdisciplinary experts in the Agency for Health Care Policy and Research (AHCPR) guidelines development, research design, literature review, law, clinical assessment, and clinical chiropractic.

Guidelines Development Process

In harmony with these general principles, the CCP has created a multidisciplinary panel, supported by staff, and led by a project director. The guidelines were produced with input from methodologists familiar with guidelines development.

The first endeavor of the panel was to analyze available scientific evidence revolving around a model which depicts the safest and most efficacious delivery of chiropractic care to the consumer. A contingent of panelists, chosen for their respective skills, directed the critical review of numerous studies and other evidence.

Since the guidelines process is one of continuing evolution, new evidence will be considered at periodic meetings to update the model of care defined by the guidelines.

The panel gathered in a second meeting to interview technique developers to ascertain the degree to which their procedures can be expressed in an evidence-based format. Individuals representing over thirty-five named techniques participated. Others made written submissions to the panel. The technique developers presented the best available evidence they had to substantiate their protocols and assessment methods.

A primary goal of the panel is to stimulate and encourage field practitioners to adapt their practices to improve patient outcomes. To achieve this objective, it was necessary to involve as many practitioners as possible in the development of workable guidelines.

Consistent with the recommendations of AHCPR, an "open forum" was held where any interested individual could participate. Practitioners offered their opinions and insights in regard to the progress of the panel. Field practitioners who were unable to attend the "open forum" session were encouraged to make written submissions. Consumer and attorney participants offered their input. A meeting was held with chiropractic consultants to secure their participation.

After sorting and evaluating the evidence gathered in the literature review, technique forum, written comments, and open forum, the initial draft of the guidelines was prepared. It was distributed to the panel for review and criticism. A revised draft was prepared based upon this input.

International input from the field was obtained when the working draft guidelines documents was submitted to 195 peer reviewers in 12 countries.

After incorporation of the suggestions of the reviewers, a final draft was presented to the panel for approval. This document was then submitted for proofreading and typesetting.

The purpose of these guidelines is to provide the doctor of chiropractic with a "user friendly" compendium of recommendations based upon the best available evidence. It is designed to facilitate, not replace, clinical judgment.

As Sackett wrote, "External clinical evidence can inform, but can never replace, individual clinical expertise, and it is this expertise that decides whether the external evidence applies to the individual patient at all and, if so, how it should be integrated into a clinical decision. Similarly, any external guideline must be integrated with individual clinical expertise in deciding whether and how it matches the patient's clinical state, predicament, and preferences, and thereby whether it should be applied." [1]

The most compelling reason for creating, disseminating, and utilizing clinical practice guidelines is to improve the quality of health care.

1. Sackett DL. Editorial: Evidence-based medicine. Spine 1998; 23(10):1085.

2. Position paper #1. Association of Chiropractic Colleges. July 1996.

Ratings and Categories of Evidence

Ratings

Established. Accepted as appropriate for use in chiropractic practice for the indications and applications stated.

Investigational. Further study is warranted. Evidence is equivocal, or insufficient to justify a rating of "established."

Inappropriate. Insufficient favorable evidence exists to support the use of this procedure in chiropractic practice.

Categories of Evidence

E: Expert opinion based on clinical experience, basic science rationale, and/or individual case studies. Where appropriate, this category includes legal opinions.

L: Literature support in the form of reliability and validity studies, observational studies, "pre-post" studies, and/or multiple case studies. Where appropriate, this category includes case law.

C: Controlled studies, including randomized and non-randomized clinical trials of acceptable quality.

Disclaimer

These guidelines are for informational purposes. Utilization of these guidelines is voluntary. They are not intended to replace the clinical judgement of the chiropractor. It is acknowledged that alternative practices are possible and may be preferable under certain clinical conditions. The appropriateness of a given procedure must be determined by the judgement of the practitioner and the needs and preferences of the individual patient.

It is not the purpose or intent of these guidelines to provide legal advice, or to supplant any statutes, rules, and regulations of a government body having jurisdiction over the practice of chiropractic.

These guidelines address vertebral subluxation in chiropractic practice, and do not purport to include all procedures which are permitted by law in the practice of chiropractic. Lack of inclusion of a procedure in these guidelines does not necessarily mean that the procedure is inappropriate for use in the practice of chiropractic.

Participation in the guidelines development process does not necessarily imply agreement with the final product. This includes persons who participated in the technique conference, leadership conference, open forum, and peer review process. Listing of names acknowledge participation only, not necessarily approval or endorsement.

The guidelines reflect the consensus of the panel, which gave final approval to the recommendations.

1 History and Chiropractic Examination

CASE HISTORY

RECOMMENDATION

A thorough case history should precede the initiation of chiropractic care. The elements of this history should include general information, reason for seeking chiropractic care, onset and duration of any symptomatic problem, family history, past health history, occupational history, and social history.
Rating: Established
Evidence: E, L

Commentary

The purpose of the case history is to elicit information which might reveal salient points concerning the patient's spinal and general health that may lead the chiropractor to elect appropriate examination procedures. The case history may provide information which will assist the chiropractor in determining the safety and appropriateness of chiropractic care as well as the nature of additional analytical procedures to be performed. History taking is considered a key element of quality patient care necessary for effective doctor-patient communication and improved patient health outcomes.[1-4] Verbal, nonverbal and cognitive assessment are also included in the patient history. The chiropractic case history should emphasize eliciting information relevant to the etiology and clinical manifestations of vertebral subluxation.

CHIROPRACTIC EXAMINATION

RECOMMENDATION

The initial chiropractic examination shall include a case history and an assessment for the presence of vertebral subluxation, which, if present, is to be noted with regard to location and character. A review of systems may be conducted at the discretion of the practitioner, consistent with individual training and applicable state laws.

Reassessments may be conducted periodically throughout a course of chiropractic care to assess patient progress. Such reassessments typically emphasize re-examination of findings which were positive on the previous examination, although need not be limited to same. Reassessment is also indicated in the case of trauma or change in the clinical status of a patient.
Rating: Established
Evidence: E, L

Commentary

The term subluxation has a long history in the healing arts literature. It may be used differently outside of the chiropractic profession. The earliest non-chiropractic English definition is attributed to Randall Holme in 1668. Holme defined subluxation as "a dislocation or putting out of joynt"[5] In medical literature, subluxation often refers to an osseous disrelationship which is less than a dislocation.[6] However, B.J. Palmer, the developer of chiropractic, hypothesized that the "vertebral subluxation" was unique from the medical use of the term "subluxation" in that it also interfered with the transmission of neurological information independent of what has come to be recognized as the action potential. Since this component has yet to be identified in a quantitative sense, practitioners currently assess the presence and correction of vertebral subluxation through parameters which measure its other components.[7] These may include some type of vertebral biomechanical abnormality,[8-14] soft tissue insult of the spinal cord and/or associated structures[15-49] and some form of neurological dysfunction involving the synapse separate from the transmission of neurological information referred to by Palmer.[50-57]

As noted, chiropractic definitions of subluxation include a neurological component. In this regard, Lantz [58] stated "common to all concepts of subluxation are some form of kinesiologic[al...sic] dysfunction and some form of neurologic[al...sic] involvement." In a recently adopted position paper, The Association of Chiropractic Colleges accepted a definition of subluxation as follows: "A subluxation is a complex of functional and/or structural and/or pathological articular changes that compromise neural integrity and may influence organ system function and general health."[59] The case history and examination are means of acquiring information pertinent to the location and analysis of subluxation. This information is primarily used to characterize subluxation regarding its presence, location, duration, and type. Additionally, the information gained through analysis guides the practitioner to ascertain which chiropractic techniques best suit the patient to effect correction of the condition.

Data collected during the patient's initial consultation and examination, pertaining to the health history and presenting concerns, thus supports the decision-making process of the practitioner. This information, relayed by the practitioner to the patient, further serves to incorporate the patient into the decision-making process regarding chiropractic care.

Elements of the Examination

History

Important elements of the case history include previous and present social and occupational events revealed by the patient; unusual sensations, moods or actions relative to the patient, with dates of occurrence and duration; previous chiropractic and non-chiropractic intervention; and other factors. The case history usually includes the following:

1. Patient clinical profile.
    A. Age.
    B. Gender.
    C. Occupation.
    D. Other information germane to the presenting complaint, if any.

2. Primary reasons for seeking chiropractic care.
    A. Primary reason.
    B. Secondary reason.
    C. Other factors contributing to the primary and secondary reasons.

3. Chief complaint, if one exists. This may include onset and duration of symptoms as well as their subjective and objective characteristics, and location, as well as aggravating or relieving factors.
    A Trauma, by etiology, when possible.
    B. Chief complaint.
    C. Characteristics of chief complaint.
    D. Intensity/frequency/location, radiation/onset/duration.
    E. Aggravating/arresting factors.
    F. Previous interventions (including chiropractic care), treatments, medications, surgery.
    G. Quality of pain, if present.
    H. Sleeping position and sleep patterns.

4. Family history.
    A. Associated health problems of relatives.
    B. Cause of parents' or siblings' death and age of death.

5. Past health history.
    A. Overall health status.
    B. Previous illnesses.
    C. Surgery.
    D. Previous injury or trauma.
    E. Medication and reactions.
    F. Allergies.
    G. Pregnancies and outcomes.
    H. Substance abuse and outcomes.

6. Social and occupational history.
    A. Level of education.
    B. Job description.
    C. Work schedule.
    D. Recreational activities.
    E. Lifestyle (hobbies, level of exercise, drug use, nature of diet).
    F. Psychosocial and mental health.

Chiropractic Analysis

Complementing the case history is the necessity of conducting a thorough chiropractic analysis. This involves procedures which indicate the presence, location, and character of vertebral subluxation. Inherent in this process is the noting of unusual findings, both related and unrelated to vertebral subluxation. This information is useful in determining the safety and appropriateness of chiropractic care.

The analysis is based partly upon the recognition that vertebral subluxation may be asymptomatic, yet still exert various physiological effects. Thus, by assimilating information relative to certain body systems, the presence of vertebral subluxation may be inferred. Examination protocols have been developed by field practitioners and researchers. Many of these protocols have been deemed acceptable by the various chiropractic educational institutions. This acceptance is expressed either through adding the protocols to the curriculum, or awarding continuing education credit to post-graduate seminars instructing these protocols, thus judging them to be sufficient in safety, efficacy, and validity to be included in clinical practice.

Manual palpation is a basic element of the chiropractic examination. This aspect of analysis includes palpation of the bony elements of the spine and includes assessment of the motion of the spine as a whole as well as the individual vertebral motion segments. Palpation of the numerous muscles which attach to and control the stability, posture, and motion of the spine is included. Static vertebral position is analyzed for abnormality. The chiropractor is additionally interested in locating areas of abnormal segmental motion to identify hypermobile segments and segments with decreased joint play (hypomobility). Palpation may also include evaluation of soft tissue compliance, tenderness, and asymmetric or hypertonic muscle contraction. The presence of vertebral subluxation may bring with it varying degrees of attendant edema, capsulitis, muscle splinting, and tenderness to digital palpation. There may be tenderness of the spinous processes upon percussion of these structures when vertebral subluxation is present.

Neurological components of the subluxation, postural distortions and other factors may bring deep and superficial myospasm to muscles of the spine, pelvis and extremities. Palpation may reveal myofascial trigger points which are associated with the articular dysfunctions accompanying vertebral subluxations. Muscular involvement may manifest as "taut and tender" fibers.

Visual inspection of the spine and paraspinal region may reveal areas of hypo- or hyperemia associated with vertebral subluxation. Observation of patient posture is an important element of chiropractic analysis.[60-62] Posture has far-reaching effects on physiology, biomechanics, psychology, and esthetics.[63] Proper body alignment relates to functional efficiency while poor structural alignment limits function. Changes in posture are considered in some chiropractic approaches as a measure of outcome.[64-69] Plain film radiographs, as well as other forms of imaging may provide information concerning the integrity of osseous and soft tissues as well as juxtapositional relationships. Other assessments such as leg length analysis,[70-94] palpatory and strength challenges[95-130] are also employed to assess states of muscular responses to neurological facilitation. Spinal distortions and resultant neurological interference may create postural or neurological reflex syndromes which result in a functional change in apparent leg length. This information is also combined with skin temperature assessments[131-138] and/or electromyography[139-167, 175-180] as well as technique-specific examination procedures to evaluate the integrity of the nervous system.[181-182] Although clinical tradition supports the use of orthopedic and neurological tests in chiropractic practice, research to support the applicability of many of these tests to the assessment of vertebral subluxation is lacking or negative.[168-174] Orthopedic and neurological tests are indicated only when relevant to the assessment of vertebral subluxation, or when determining the safety and appropriateness of chiropractic care.

It is recognized that research will continue to evolve the most efficacious applications of assessment techniques described in this document. However, the literature is sufficiently supportive of their usefulness in regard to the chiropractic examination to warrant inclusion as components of the present recommendation.

The chiropractic examination may include, but not be limited to:

1. Clinical examination procedures.
   A. Palpation (static osseous and muscular, motion).
   B. Range of motion.
   C. Postural examination.
   D. Muscle strength testing.
   E. Orthopedic/neurological tests.
   F. Mental status examination procedures.
   G. Quality of life assessment instruments.
   H. Substance abuse and outcomes.

2. Imaging and instrumentation
   A. Plain film radiography.
   B. Videofluoroscopy.
   C. Computerized tomography.
   D. Magnetic resonance imaging.
   E. Range of motion.
   F. Thermography.
   G. Temperature reading instruments.
   H. Electromyography.
   I. Pressure algometry.
   J. Nerve/function tests.
   K. Electroencephalography.

3. Review of systems.
   A. Musculoskeletal.
   B. Cardiovascular and respiratory.
   C. Gastrointestinal.
   D. Genitourinary.
   E. Nervous system.
   F. Eye, ear, nose and throat.
   G. Endocrine.

Clinical Impression

An appropriate interpretation of case history and examination findings is essential in determining the appropriate application of chiropractic care within the overall needs of the patient. The clinical impression derived from patient information acquired through the examination process is ultimately translated into a plan of corrective care, including those elements which are contraindicated. The clinical impression serves to focus the practitioner on the patient's immediate and long-term needs. It is through this process that a clear picture is created regarding the patient's status relative to chiropractic care.

Initial Consultation

The initial consultation serves the purpose of determining how chiropractic care can benefit the patient. It is during this interchange that the practitioner presents and discusses examination findings with the patient. Additionally, during the initial consultation, the practitioner should take the opportunity to present his/her practice objectives and terms of acceptance. The terms of acceptance provides the patient with information regarding the objectives, responsibilities and limitations of the care to be provided by the practitioner. This reciprocal acknowledgment allows both practitioner and patient to proceed into the plan of care with well-defined expectations.

While not limited to the following, it is suggested that the initial consultation include the following parameters:

1. Description of chiropractic: Chiropractic is a primary contact health care profession receiving patients without necessity of referral from other health care providers. Traditionally, chiropractic focuses on the anatomy of the spine and its immediate articulations, the existence and nature of vertebral subluxation, and a scope of practice which encompasses the correction of vertebral subluxation, as well as educating and advising patients concerning this condition, and its impact on general health.

2. Professional responsibility: To assess the propriety of applying methods of analysis and vertebral subluxation correction to patients; to recognize and deal appropriately with emergency situations; and to report to the patient any nonchiropractic findings discovered during the course of the examination, making referral to other health professionals for care or for evaluation of conditions outside the scope of chiropractic practice. Such referral does not obviate the responsibility of the chiropractor for providing appropriate chiropractic care.

3. Practice objective: The professional practice objective of the chiropractor is to correct or stabilize the vertebral subluxation in a safe and effective manner. The correction of vertebral subluxation is not considered a specific cure or treatment for any specific medical disease or symptom. Rather, it is applicable to any patient exhibiting vertebral subluxation, regardless of the presence or absence of symptoms and diseases.

References

1. Bates B. A guide to physical examination. Lippincott, Philadelphia, PA. 1982.

2. Saad M. Medical history taking records and forms control. J Can Chiro Assoc 1988. ·

3. Strachan G. Chiropractic physician records: essential for defense and new practice areas. DC Tracts 1990; 2(6)315-321.

4. Vernon H. Clinical Note: S.O.R.E. A record keeping system for chiropractic treatment visits. J Can Chiro Assoc 1990:34(2)93.

5. Holme R. Academy of Armory. Menston, England: Published by the Author in 1688. Reprinted by the Scholar Press, Ltd., 1972.

6. Stedman TL. Stedman's Medical Dictionary (26th Ed.). Baltimore, Williams & Wilkins, 1995.

7. Palmer BJ. The subluxation specific - the adjustment specific. Davenport: The Palmer School of Chiropractic, 1934 (1986 printing):15.

8. Ito J, Tadano S, Neda K. A biomechanical definition of spinal segmental instability taking personal and disc level differences into account. Spine 1993; 18(15): 2295-2304.

9. Kawchuk G, Herzog W. Biomechanical characterization (Fingerprinting) of five novel methods of cervical spine manipulation. J Manipulative Physiol Ther 1993; 16(9): 573-577.

10. Kondracki M, Weston J, Breen K. A comparison between the 3-space isotrak and digital videofluoroscopy in the assessment of lumbar flexion. Proc of the Int'l Conf on Spinal Manip 1994; 95.

11. Mawhiney R. Clinical Report: reduction of minor lumbar scoliosis in a 57-year-old female. J Chiro Research 1989; 2:48-51.

12. Mawhiney R. Vertebral median line angle and vertebral/pelvic measurements versus Cobb's angle in chiropractic evaluation of scoliosis. Chiropractic: J Chiro Research and Clinical Investigation. 1991; 7(1):10-15.

13. Zengel F, Davis B. Biomechanical analysis by chiropractic radiography: Part II. Effects of x-ray projectional distortion on apparent vertebral rotation. J Manipulative Physiol Ther 1988; 11(5): 380-389.

14. Zengel F, Davis B. Biomechanical analysis by chiropractic radiography: Part I A simple method for determining x-ray projectional distortion. J Manipulative Physiol Ther 1988; 11(4): 273-280.

15. Antos J, Robinson K, Keating J, et al. Interrater reliability of fluoroscopic detection of fixation in the mid-cervical spine. Chiropractic Technique 1990; 2(2): 53-55.

16. Brand N, Gizoni C. Moiré contourography and infrared thermography: changes resulting from chiropractic adjustments. J Manipulative Physiol Ther 1982; 5:113-116.

17. Brightbill T, Pile N, Eichelberger R, et al. Normal magnetic resonance imaging and abnormal discography in lumbar disc disruption. Spine 1994; 19(9):1075-1077.

18. Brodeur R, Hansmeier D. Variability of intervertebral angle calculations for lateral cervical videofluoroscopic examinations. Proc of the Int'l Conf on Spinal Manip 1993; 37.

19. Byrd R, Kahler J, Leaman S, et al. Reliability of magnetic resonance imaging for morphometry of the intervertebral foramen. Proc of the Int'l Conf on Spinal Manip 1990; 79-82.

20. Cantu J, Cramer G, Dorsett R, et al. Magnetic resonance imaging of the cervical intervertebral foramina: comparison of two techniques. Proc of the Int'l Conf on Spinal Manip 1994; 101-103.

21. Cramer G, Cantu J, Greenstein J, et al. The accuracy of magnetic resonance imaging in determining the vertical dimensions of the cervical intervertebral foramina. Proc of the Int'l Conf on Spinal Manip 1993; 38-40.

22. Cramer G, Howe J, Glenn W, et al. Comparison of computed tomography to magnetic resonance imaging in evaluation of the intervertebral foramen. The National College of Chiropractic, Lombard, IL, Los Angeles College of Chiropractic Whittier, CA, Private Practice of Medical Radiology, Carson, CA, Computer programmer, Los Angeles, CA.

23. Cramer G., Howe J, Glenn W, et al. Lumbar intervertebral foramen dimensions from thirty-seven human subjects as determined by magnetic resonance imaging. Proc of the Int'l Conf on Spinal Manip 1992; 3-5.

24. Daruwalla J, Balasubramaniam P. Moiré topography in scoliosis—its accuracy in detecting the site and size of the curve. J Bone Joint Surg 1985; 67:211-213.

25. Bennett SF, Hayde TN. Cervical spondylolisthesis: a case report. ACA J Chiro. 1991; 2:69-71.

26. Denton T, Randall F, Deinlein D. The use of instant moiré photographs to reduce exposure from scoliosis radiographs. Spine 1992; 17(5):509-512.

27. EilBert L, Spector B. The moiré contourographic analysis controversy: A question of validity in present-day clinical practice. J Manipulative Physiol Ther 1979; 2:85.

28. Eldevik O, Dugstad G, Orrison W, et al. The effect of clinical bias on the interpretation of myelography and spinal computed tomography. Radiology 1982; 145:85-89.

29. Gertzbein S, Holtby R, Tile M, et al. Determination of a locus of instantaneous centers of rotation of the lumbar disc by moiré fringes. A new technique. Spine 1984; 9:409-413.

30. Gertzbein S, Seligman J, Holtby R, et al. Centrode patterns and segmental instability in degenerative disc disease. Spine 1985; 10(3):257-261.

31. Ho E, Upadhyay S, Chan F, et al. New methods of measuring vertebral rotation from computed tomographic scans. An intraobserver and interobserver study on girls with scoliosis. Spine 1993; 18(9):1173-1177.

32. Laulund T, Sojbjerg J, Horlyck E. Moiré topography in school screening for structural scoliosis. ACTA Orthop Scand 1982; 53:765-768.

33. Leung, S. The value of cineradiographic motion studies in the diagnosis of dysfunctions of the cervical spine. Bull Eur Chiro Union 1977; 25(2):28-43.

34. Montgomery F, Persson U, Benoni G, et al. Screening for scoliosis. A cost-effectiveness analysis. Spine 1990; 15(2):67-70.

35. Pope M, Wilder D, Stokes I, et al. Biomechanical testing as an aid to decision making in low back pain patients. Spine 1979; 4(2):135-140.

36. Reinke T, Jahn W. Spinal diagnostic imaging: computerized axial tomography vs. magnetic resonance imaging. Am J Chiro Med 1988; 1(14):181-184.

37. Ruggerone M, Austin J. Moiré topography in scoliosis: correlations with vertebral lateral curvature as determined by radiography. Phys Ther 1986; 66(7):1072-1077.

38. Sahlstrand, T. The clinical value of moiré topography in the management of scoliosis. Spine 1986; 11:409-417.

39. Spector B, Eilbert L, Finando S, et al. Video integrated measurement system. J Manipulative Physiol Ther 1982; 5(2): 55-61.

40. Spector B, Eilbert L, Fukuda F, et al. Development and application of specteil indices for quantitative analysis in moiré contourography. J Manipulative Physiol Ther 1979; 2(1):16-25

41. Spector B, Finando S, Fukuda F, et al. An intergrated video biofeedback/moiré system for diagnosis and treatment: A preliminary report. J Manipulative Physiol Ther 1980; 3(4):220-224.

42. Spector B, Fukuda F, Krammer L, Thorschmidt E. A preliminary integrated video biofeedback/moiré system. Am Chiro 1981; 14, 19.

43. Stokes I, Moreland M. Concordance of back surface asymmetry and spine shape in idiopathic scoliosis. Spine 1989; 14(1):73-78.

44. Tibbles A, Belanger M, Grinder L, et al. Moiré topography in scoliosis screening: A study of the precision of the method. Proc of the Int'l Conf on Spinal Manip 1991; 43-44.

45. Turner-Smith A, Harris J, Houghton G, Jefferson R. A method for analysis of back shape in scoliosis. J Biomech 1988; 21:497-509.

46. Van Wijk, M. Moiré contourograph: An accuracy analysis. J Biomech 1980; 13:605-613.

47. Wallace H, Wagon R, Pierce W. Inter-examiner reliability using videofluoroscope to measure cervical spine kinematics: A sagittal plane (lateral view). Proc of the Int'l Conf on Spinal Manip 1992; 7-8.

48. Willner, S. A comparative study of the efficiency of different types of school screening for scoliosis. ACTA Orthop Scand 1982; 53:769-774.

49. Willner, S. Prevalence study of trunk asymmetries structural scoliosis in 10-year-old school children. Spine 1984; 9:644-647.

50. Bamford C, Graeme K. Percutaneous S1 root somatosensory evoked potential. Electromyogr Clin Neurophysiol 1995; 35:181-186.

51. Chistyakov A, Soustiel J, Hafner H, et al. Motor and somatosensory conduction in cervical myelopathy and radiculopathy. Spine 1995; 20(19):2135-3140.

52. Collins K, Pfleger B. The neurophysiological evaluation of the subluxation complex: documenting the neurological component with somatosensory evoked potentials. CRJ 1994; 3(1): 40-48.

53. Glick, D. Characterization of neurological insult in the low back utilizing somatosensory evoked potential studies. Proc of the Int'l Conf on Spinal Manip 1994; 17.

54. Kai Y, Owen J, Allen B, et al. Relationship between evoked potentials and clinical status in spinal cord ischemia. Spine 1994; 19(10):1162-1168.

55. Leppanen R, Maguire J, Wallace S, et al. Intraoperative lower extremity reflex muscle activity as an adjunct to conventional somatosensory-evoked potentials and descending neurogenic monitoring in idiopathic. Spine 1995; 20(17):1872-1877.

56. Swenson, R. Dermatomal somatosensory evoked potentials: A review of the literature. Journal of the Neuromusculoskeletal System 1994; 2(2):45-51.

57. Zhu Y, Hsieh C, Haldeman S, et al. Paraspinal muscle somatosensory evoked potentials in low back pain patients with muscle spasm: A quantitative study of the effect of spinal manipulation. Proc of the Int'l Conf on Spinal Manip 1994; 16.

58. Lantz CA. The vertebral subluxation concept. In: Gatterman MI, ed. Foundation of Chiropractic Subluxation. St. Louis, MO: Mosby, 1995.

59. Association of Chiropractic Colleges (ACC) Position on Chiropractic; Position paper #1; July 1996; <http://Lifenet.life.edu/other/acc.html>

60. Adams A, Lopez D, Wild S, et al. Intra- and inter-examiner reliability of plumb line posture analysis measurements using a three dimensional electro-goniometer. Res For 1988; 4(3):60-72.

61. Ebrall, P. An estimation of the clinical error for the metrecom computer-assisted goniometer. Chiropractic Technique 1993; 5(1):1-4.

62. McGregor M, Mior S. Anatomical and functional perspectives of the cervical spine: Part 1: the "normal" cervical spine. JCCA 1989; 33(3):123-9.

63. Gill-Body K, Krebs D. Usefulness of biomechanical measurement approaches in rehabilitation. Topics in Geriatric Rehabilitation 1994; 10(2):82-96.

64. Leach RA. The chiropractic theories. A symposia of chiropractic research. Baltimore: Williams & Wilkins, 1986; 35-46.

65. Decosta, A. The correction of lumbosacral and sacroiliac disrelationships. Digest Chiro Econ 1983; 26(3):14-19, 140-143.

66. Keating, J. Technique system application: The Gonstead approach. J Chiro Tech 1991; 3(3): 135-136.

67. Lopes M, Plaugher G, Ray S. Closed reduction of lumbar retrolisthesis: A report of two cases. Proc of the Int'l Conf on Spinal Manip (Wash D.C.) 1991; 110-114.

68. Maltezopoulos V, Armitage N. A comparison of four chiropractic systems in the diagnosis of sacroiliac malfunction. Euro J Chiro 1984; 32(1):4-42..

69. Nansel D, Cremata E, Carlson J, et al. Effect of unilateral spinal adjustments on goniometrically-assessed cervical lateral-flexion end-range asymmetries in otherwise asymptomatic subjects. J Manipulative Physiol Ther 1989; 12(6):419-427.

70. Beattie P, Isaacson K, Riddle D, et al. Validity of derived measurements of leg-length differences obtained by use of a tape measure. Phys Ther 1990; 70(3):150-157.

71. Bowman C, Gribble R. The value of the forward flexion test and three tests of leg length changes in the clinical assessment of movement of the sacroiliac joint. Journal of Orthopaedic Medicine 1995; 17(2):66-67.

72. Burke M, Rhudy T. Inter-examiner reliability of functional leg-length assessment. Am J Chiro Med 1990; 3(2):63-66.

73. Giles LGF, Taylor JR. Low-back pain associated with leg length inequality. Spine 1981; 6:510-521.

74. Deboer K, Harmon R, Savoie S, et al. Inter- and intra-examiner reliability of leg length differential measurement: A preliminary study. J Manipulative Physiol Ther 1983; 9(2):61-66.

75. Dewitt J, Osterbauer P, Stelmach G, et al. Optoelectric measurement of leg length changes during isolation tests. Transactions of the Consortium for Chiropractic Research 1993; 8:156-157.

76. Dewitt J, Osterbauer P, Stelmach G. Optoelectric measurement of changes in leg length inequality resulting from isolation tests. J Manipulative Physiol Ther 1994; 17(8):530-538.

77. Falltrick D, Pierson S. Precise measurement of functional leg length inequality and changes due to cervical spine rotation in pain-free students. J Manipulative Physiol Ther 1989; 12(5):364-368.

78. Frogley, H. The value and validity of the leg check as used in the chiropractic profession. Dig Chiro Econ 1987; 29(5):24-25.

79. Fuhr A, Osterbauer P. A preliminary look at inter-examiner reliability of prone leg lengths. Proc of the Int'l Conf on Spinal Manip 1989; 213-218.

80. Fuhr A, Osterbauer P. Interexaminer reliability of relative leg-length evaluations in the prone, extended position. Chiro Tech 1989; 1(1):13-18.

81. Haas M, Peterson D, Panzer D, et al. Reactivity of leg alignment to articular pressure testing: Evaluation of a diagnostic test using a randomized crossover clinical trial approach. J Manipulative Physiol Ther 1993; 16(4):220-227.

82. Haas M, Peterson D, Rothman E, et al. Responsiveness of leg alignment changes associated with articular pressure testing to spinal manipulation: The use of a randomized clinical trial design to evaluate. J Manipulative Physiol Ther 1993; 16(5):306-311.

83. Haas M, Peterson D, Solomon S, et al. Reactivity of leg length to articular pressure testing: A randomized cross-over clinical trial. Proc of the Int'l Conf on Spinal Manip 1992; 121-122.

84. Haas M. Inter- and intra-examiner reliability of leg-length differential measurement: A preliminary study. J Manipulative Physiol Ther 1988; 11(1):50-51.

85. Lawrence D. Chiropractic concepts of the short leg: A critical review. J Manipulative Physiol Ther 1985; 8(3):157-161.

86. Mannello D. Leg length inequality: A literature review. Transactions of the Consortium for Chiropractic Research 1992; 7:67-92.

87. Montgomery D, Egan I, Pollard H. Palpable unilateral sacral prominence as a clinical sign of lower limb anisomelia: A pilot study. J Manipulative Physiol Ther 1995; 18(6):353-356.

88. Mootz R, Hansen D, Adams A. The value of leg length inequality and specific contact short lever adjusting in chiropractic practice: Results of a consensus process by chiropractic expert panels. Chiro Tech 1993; 5(1):26-31.

89. Rhodes D, Mansfield E, Bishop P, et al. Comparison of leg length inequality methods as estimators of the femur head height difference on standing x-ray. J Manipulative Physiol Ther 1995; 18(7):448-452.

90. Rhodes D, Mansfield E, Bishop P. The validity of the prone leg check as an estimate of standing leg length inequality measured by x-ray. J Manipulative Physiol Ther 1995; 18(6):343-346.

91. Rock B. Short leg—A review and survey. J Aust Chiro Assoc 1988; 18(3):91-96.

92 Shambaugh P, Sclafani L, Fanselow D. Reliability of the Derifield-Thompson test for leg length inequality, and use of the test to demonstrate cervical adjusting efficacy. J Manipulative Physiol Ther 1988; 11(5):396-399.

93. Troyanovich, S. Letters to the editor: optoelectric measurement of changes of leg length inequality resulting from isolation tests. J Manipulative Physiol Ther 1995; 18(5):322.

94. Venn E, Wakefield K, Thompson P. A comparative study of leg length checks. Eur J Chiro 1983; 31(2):68-80.

95. Bendtsen L, Jensen R. Pressure-controlled palpation: A new technique which increases the reliability of manual palpation. CEPHDF 1995; 15:205-210.

96. Bergstrom E, Courtis G. An inter- intra-examiner reliability study of motion palpation of the lumbar spine in lateral flexion in the seated position. Eur J Chiro 1986; 34(3):121-141.

97. Boline P, Keating J, Brist J, et al. Interexaminer reliability of palpatory evaluations of the lumbar spine. Am J Chiro Med 1988; 1(1):5-11.

98. Breen A. The reliability of palpation and other diagnostic methods. J Manipulative Physiol Ther 1992; 15(1):54-56.

99. Byfield D, Mathiasen J, Sangren C. Intra- and inter-examiner reliability of static palpation of specific landmarks in the lumbar spine and pelvis using an invisible skin marking pen. Proc of the World Chiro Congress 1991.

100. Byfield D. Intra- and inter-examiner reliability of body landmark identification in the lumbar spine. Eur J Chiro 1992; 72:13-17.

101. Byfield D. Preliminary studies with a mechanical model for the evaluation of spinal motion palpation in the lumbar spine. Proc of the Int'l Conf on Spinal Manip 1990; 215-218.

102. Carmichael J. Inter- and intra-examiner reliability of palpation for sacroiliac joint dysfunction. J Manipulative Physiol Ther 1987; 10(4):164-171.

103. Cassidy J. Sacroiliac motion palpation. JCCA 1980; 24(4):143.

104. Cooperstein R, Gardner R, Nansel D. Concordance of two methods of motion palpation with goniometrically-assessed cervical lateral flexion asymmetry. Proc of the Int'l Conf on Spinal Manip 1991; 235-259.

105. Cooperstein R, Gardner R, Nansel D. Concordance of two methods of motion palpation with goniometrically-assessed cervical lateral flexion asymmetry. Palmer College of Chiropractic West, Sunnyvale, CA.

106. Gonnella C, Paris S, Kutner M. Reliability in evaluating passive intervertebral motion. Phys Ther 1982; 62(4):436-444.

107. Haas M, Nyiendo J. Interexaminer concordance in detecting joint-play asymmetries in the cervical spines of otherwise asymptomatic subjects. J Manipulative Physiol Ther 1990; 13(6):346-348.

108. Harvey D, Byfield D. Preliminary studies with a mechanical model for the evaluation of spinal motion palpation. Clinical Biomechanics 1991; 6(2):79-82.

109. Herzog W, Read L, Conway P, et al. Reliability of motion palpation procedures to detect sacroiliac joint fixations. J Manipulative Physiol Ther 1989; 12(2):86-92.

110. Jensen KJ, Gemmell H, Thiel H. Motion palpation accuracy using a mechanical spinal model. Eur J Chiro 1993; 41:67-73.

111. Johnston W, Allan B, Hendra J, et al. Interexaminer study of palpation in detecting location of spinal segmental dysfunction. J Am Osteopath Assoc 1983; 82(11):839-845.

112. Johnston W, Beal M, Blum G. Passive gross motion testing: Part 3. examiner agreement on selected subjects. J Am Osteopath Assoc 1982; 82(5):309-313.

113. Johnston W. The role of static and motion palpation in structural diagnosis. J Am Osteopath Assoc 1975; 75:421-424.

114. Keating J. Inter-examiner reliability of motion palpation of the lumbar spine: A review of quantitative literature. Am J Chiro Med 1989; 2(3):107-110.

115. Keating J. Interexaminer reliability of motion palpation of the lumbar spine: A review of the quantitative literature. J Manipulative Physiol Ther 1990; 13(1):55.

116. Kilgore W. Interexaminer reliability of palpatory evaluation of the lumbar spine. Am J Chiro Med 1988; 1(3):142.

117. King R, Warner A, Lapierre P. Student interexaminer reliability in localization of hypomobile joints of the spine utilizing motion palpation techniques. International Review of Chiropractic (ICA Review) 1981; 35(2):39-40.

118. Lewitt K, Liebenson C. Palpation problems and implications. J Manipulative Physiol Ther 1993; 16(9):586-590.

119. Love R. Inter- and intra-examiner reliability of motion palpation for the thoracolumbar spine. J Manipulative Physiol Ther 1987; 10:1-4.

120. Mior S, King R, McGregor M, et al. Intra and interexaminer reliability of motion palpation in the cervical spine. JCCA 1985; 29:195-199.

121. Mootz R, Keating J, Kontz H, et al. Intra- and interobserver reliability of passive motion palpation of the lumbar spine. J Manipulative Physiol Ther 1989; 12(6):440-445.

122. Nansel D, Peneff A, Jansen R, et al. Inter-examiner concordance in detecting joint-play asymmetries in the cervical spines of otherwise asymptomatic subjects. J Manipulative Physiol Ther 1989; 12(6):428-433.

123. Panzer D. Lumbar motion palpation: A literature review. Transactions of the Consortium for Chiropractic Research 1991; 171-186.

124. Panzer D. The reliability of lumbar motion palpation. J Manipulative Physiol Ther 1992; 15(8):518-524.

125. Paydar D, Thiel H, Gemmell H. Intra- and interexaminer reliability of certain pelvic palpatory procedures and the sitting flexion test for sacroiliac joint mobility and dysfunction. Journal of the Neuromusculoskeletal System 1994; 2(2):65-69.

126. Ray S. The Gonstead system of lumbar motion palpation. Transactions of the Consortium for Chiropractic Research 1991; 162-163.

127. Russell R. Diagnostic palpation of the spine: A review of procedures and assessment of their reliability. J Manipulative Physiol Ther 1983; 6(4):181-183.

128. Vernon H, Aker P, Menko M, et al. Evaluation of neck muscle strength with a modified sphygmomanometer dynamometer: reliability and validity. J Manipulative Physiol Ther. 1992, 15(6):343-9.

129. Hyytiainen K, Salminen J, Suvitie T, et al. Reproducibility of nine tests to measure spinal mobility and trunk muscle strength. Scand J Rehabil Med. 1991; 23:3-10.

130. Wiles M. Reproducibility and interexaminer correlation of motion palpation findings of the sacroiliac joints. JCCA 1980; 24(2):56-69.

131. Uematsu S, Haberman J, Pochaczevsky R, et al. Thermography as a diagnostic aid in sciatica: a commentary on experimental methods, data interpretation and conclusions. Thermology. 1985; 1(1):43-50.

132. Brand N, Gizoni C. Moiré contourography and infrared thermography: changes resulting from chiropractic adjustments. J Manipulative Physiol Ther 1982; 5:113-6

133. Diakow P. The status of thermography as a diagnostic tool. J Manipulative Physiol Ther 1990; 13(2):121.

134. Ebrall P, Iggo A, Hobson P, et al. Preliminary report: the thermal characteristics of spinal levels identified as having different temperature by contact thermocouple measurement (nervo scope). Chiropr J Aust 1994; 24:139-146.

135. Hart J. Skin temperature patterns of the posterior neck used in chiropractic analysis- A Case Study. Chiropractic 1991; 7(2):46-8

136. Kobrossi T. L5 and S1 nerve fiber irritation demonstrated by liquid crystal thermography-a case report. JCCA 1985; 29:199-202.

137. Schram S, Hosek R, Owens E. Computerized paraspinal skin surface temperature scanninng: a technical report. J Manipulative Physiol Ther 1982; 5(3)117-21.

138. Wallace H, Wallace J, Resh R. Advances in paraspinal thermographic analysis. Chiropractic Research Journal. 1993; 2(3):39-55.

139. Ahern D, Follick M, Council J, et al. Reliability of lumbar paravertebral EMG assessment in chronic low back pain. Arch Phys Med Rehab 1986; 67:762.

140. Brown WF. The physiology and technical basis of electromyography. Butterworth Publishers, Stoneham, MA,1984.

141. Calancie B, Madsen P, Lebwohl N. Stimulus-evoked EMG monitoring during transpedicular lumbosacral spine instrumentation. Spine 1994; 19(24):2780-2786.

142. Cobb C, DeVries H, Urban R, et al. Electrical activity in muscle pain. Am J Phys Med 1975; 54(2):80.

143. Andreassi JL. Psycho physiology: human behavior and physiological response. New York. Oxford University Press 1980:149-172.

144 Gentempo P, Kent C. Establishing medical necessity for paraspinal EMG scanning. Chiropractic: (J Chiro Research and Clinical Investigation) 1990; 3(1):22.

145. Kent C, Gentempo P. Static and dynamic paraspinal surface EMG: an outcome assessment for subluxation-based chiropractic care. International Review of Chiropractic. 1995; 29-35, 37.

146. Hoyt W, Hunt Jr. H, De Pauw M, et al. Electromyographic assessment of chronic low-back pain syndrome. J Am Osteopath Assoc 1981; 80(11):728-730.

147. Kent C, Fitzsimons W. Admissibility of electromyographic findings in personal injury cases. Digest Chiro Econ 1988; 30(5):43-46.

148. Kent C, Gentempo P. Medical evidence of soft tissue injury: legal aspects of paraspinal EMG findings. Am Chiro 1990; 12(12):10-15.

149. Kent C, Gentempo P. Protocol and normative data for paraspinal EMG scanning in chiropractic practice. J Chiro Research and Clinical Investigation 1990; 6(3):64-67.

150. Kent C, Hyde R. Potential applications for electromyography in chiropractic practice. Digest Chiro Econ 1987; 30(2):20-25.

151. Kent C. Surface electrode EMG/lumbar spine. Transactions of the Consortium for Chiropractic Research 1993; 8:48.

152. Komi P, Buskirk E. Reproducibility of electromyographic measurements with inserted wire electrodes and surface electrodes. Electromyography 1970; 10:357.

153. Kondo M, Matsuda H, Kureya S, et al. Electrophysiological studies of intermittent claudication in lumbar stenosis. Spine 1989; 14:862-866.

154. Konrad P, Owen J, Bridwell K. Magnetic stimulation of the spine to produce lower extremity EMG responses: significance of coil position and the presence of bone. Spine 1994; 19(24): 2812-2818.

155. Marcarian D. Factors influencing the SEMG's potential for continued future use. Transactions of the Consortium for Chiropractic Research 1993; 8:51-52.

156. Meeker W, Matheson D, Milus T, et al. Lack of correlation between scanning EMG asymmetries and history and presence of low back pain: analysis of pilot data. Proc of the Int'l Conf on Spinal Manip 1990; 230-235.

157. Meeker W, Matheson D, Wong A, et al. Lack of evidence for a relationship between low back pain and asymmetrical muscle activity using scanning electromyography. Proc of the World Chiro Congress 1991.

158. Meyer J. The current status on validity of thoracolumbar paraspinal scanning EMG as a diagnostic test: a literature review. Transactions of the Consortium for Chiropractic Research 1993; 8:21-47.

159. Meyer J. The validity of thoracolumbar paraspinal scanning EMG as a diagnostic test: an examination of the current literature. J Manipulative Physiol Ther 1994; 17(8):539-551.

160. Myerowitz M. Scanning paraspinal surface EMG: a method for corroborating post-treatment spinal and related neuromusculoskeletal symptom improvement. Journal of Occupational Rehabilitation 1994; 4(3):171-179.

161. Papakyriakou M, Triano J. Effects of filtering on the evaluation of surface EMG signals. Proc of the Int'l Conf on Spinal Manip 1993; 84.

162. Sandrini G, Antonaci F, Pucci E, et al. Comparative study with EMG, pressure alogmetry and manual palpation in tension-type headache and migraine. Cephalalgia (CEPHDF) 1994; 14:451-457.

163. Shinomiya K, Komori H, Matsuoka T, et al. Neuroradiologic and electrophysiologic assessment of cervical spondylotic amyotrophy. Spine 1994; 19(1):21-25.

164. Spector B, Eilbert L, Finando S, Fukuda F. Video integrated measurement system. J Manipulative Physiol Ther 1982; 5(2):55-61.

165. Thompson D, Biederman H. Electromyographic power spectrum analysis of the paraspinal muscles. Spine 1993; 18(15):2310-2313.

166. Triano J. Surface electrode EMG/lumbar spine: static paraspinal EMG scanning-clinical utility and validity issues. Transactions of the Consortium for Chiropractic Research 1993; 8:53-58.

167. Triano J. The validity of thoracolumbar paraspinal scanning EMG as a diagnostic test: examination of the current literature. J Manipulative Physiol Ther 1995; 18(7):482-483.

168. Strender LE, Sjoblom A, Sundell K, Ludwig R, Taube A. Interexaminer reliability in physical examination of patients with low back pain. Spine. 1997; 22(7):814-20.

169. Leamon TB. Research to reality: a critical review of the validity of various criteria for the prevention of occupationally induced low back pain disability. Ergonomics. 1994; 37(12):1959-74 0014-0139.

170. Breen A. The reliability of palpation and other diagnostic methods. J Manipulative Physiol Ther. 1992; 15(1):54-6 0161-4754.

171. Porter RW, Trailescu IF. Diurnal changes in straight leg raising. Spine. 1990; 15(2):103-6 0362-2436.

172. Nelson MA, Allen P, Clamp SE, de Dombal FT. Reliability and reproducibility of clinical findings in low-back pain. Spine. 1979; 4(2):97-101 0362-2436.

173. Potter NA, Rothstein JM. Intertester reliability for selected clinical tests of the sacroiliac joint. Phys Ther. 1985; 65(11):1671-5 0031-9023.

174. Matsumoto M, Fujimura Y, Toyama Y. Usefulness and reliability of neurological signs for level diagnosis in cervical myelopathy caused by soft disc herniation. J Spinal Disord. 1996; 9(4):317-21.

175. Kent C, Gentempo P. Static and dynamic paraspinal surface EMG: an outcome assessment for subluxation-based chiropractic care. International Review of Chiropractic. 1995; 29-35, 37.

176. Kent C, Gentempo P. Dynamic paraspinal surface EMG: a chiropractic protocol. Chiropractic Research Journal. 1993; 2(4):40-6.

177. Kent C, Gentempo P. Paraspinal EMG potentials in pediatric patients: preliminary observations. Chiropractic Research Journal. 1992; 2(2):48-52.

178. Kent C, Gentempo P. Paraspinal EMG scanning in chiropractic practice: a review. Chiropractic Research Journal. 1991; 2(1):41-9.

179. Gentempo P, Kent C, Hightower B, Minicozzi SJ. Normative data for paraspinal surface electromyographic scanning using a 25-500 Hz bandpass. Journal of Vertebral Subluxation Research. 1996; 1(1):43-46.

180. Kent C. Surface electromyography in the assessment of changes in paraspinal muscle activity associated with vertebral subluxation: a review. Journal of Vertebral Subluxation Research. 1997; 1(3):15-22.

181. Collins K, Pfleger B. The neurophysiological evaluation of subluxation complex: documenting the neurological component with somatosensory evoked potentials. Chiropractic Research Journal. 1994; 3)1):40-8.

182. Capria M. Somatosensory neurological evaluation of chiropractic manipulation. Chiropractic: J Chiro Research and Clinical Investigation 1990; 6(3):56-58.

2 Instrumentation

RECOMMENDATION

Instrumentation is indicated for the qualitative and/or quantitative assessment of the biomechanical and physiological components of vertebral subluxation. When using instrumentation, baseline values should be determined prior to the initiation of care.
Rating: Established
Evidence: E, L

Commentary

The chiropractor uses a variety of procedures to assess the vertebral subluxation. These methods may include history taking, physical examination, imaging procedures and instrumentation. Through information gained from research and personal experience, the chiropractor generally assigns a personal value to each procedure in a particular clinical circumstance. The intent of this chapter is to describe clinical applications for the various instruments that may be used by chiropractors in examining their patients for evidence of vertebral subluxation.

Definition of instrumentation: The use of any tool or device used to obtain objective data, which can be recorded in a reproducible manner, about the condition of the patient relative to vertebral subluxation. Such instrumentation as that described below may provide information concerning the biomechanical and/or neurological aspects of vertebral subluxation.

POSTURAL ANALYSIS

Sub-Recommendation

Postural analysis using plumb line devices, computerized and non-computerized instruments may be used to evaluate changes in posture associated with vertebral subluxation.
Rating: Established
Evidence: E, L

Posture analysis is recommended for determining postural aberrations associated with vertebral subluxation. The findings of such examinations should be recorded in the patient record. In order to encourage standardization of reporting, it is suggested that findings be recorded in a form consistent with manufacturers' recommendations.

Posture analysis may include the use of such devices as the plumb line, scoliometer and posturometer.[1-8] Posture is often analyzed by x-ray methods[9-13] simply by visualizing the patient and making determinations based on that visualization. The procedure is often enhanced by a plumb line and other vertical and horizontal lines.

BILATERAL AND FOUR-QUADRANT WEIGHT SCALES

Sub-Recommendation

Bilateral and four-quadrant weight scales may be used to determine the weight distribution asymmetries indicative of spinal abnormalities.
Rating: Established
Evidence: E, L

Unequal weight distribution has been shown to be indicative of spinal abnormalities.[14-18] Weight scales are a simple and effective means to determine weight distribution asymmetries.

MOIRÉ CONTOUROGRAPHY

Sub-Recommendation

Moiré contourography may be used to provide a photographic record of changes in body contour associated with vertebral subluxation.
Rating: Established
Evidence: E, L

Moiré contourography is a photographic technique which yields information regarding body contours and their variations for the purpose of evaluating structural abnormality. It is useful to the chiropractor because body surface asymmetries may be indicative of the presence of vertebral subluxation.[19-33]

INCLINOMETRY

Inclinometry may be used as a means of measuring motion against a constant vertical component of gravity as a reference. Changes in ranges of spinal motion may be associated with vertebral subluxation.
Rating: Established
Evidence: E, L

Mechanical, electronic and fluid-filled inclinometers are available.[34-38] Inclinometer measurements have been thoroughly studied regarding their ability to measure complex motions of the spine.[39-49] Inclinometers are considered superior to goniometers for assessing spinal motion.[50] Inclinometers have been shown to be accurate within 10% of those obtained by radiographic evaluation.[51] Achieving acceptable reliability is dependent upon use of standardized procedures.

GONIOMETRY

Sub-Recommendation

Goniometry, computer associated or not, may be used to measure joint motion. Inclinometry is superior to goniometry when standardized procedures are employed.

Rating: Established
Evidence: E, L

A goniometer is a protractor that may be held in the proximity of the area being measured to provide a means by which to determine degrees of motion.[35] Although goniometry is common, a wide range of variance has been reported, [56-59] expressing up to 10°-15° error.[60, 61]

ALGOMETRY

Sub-Recommendation

Algometry may be used to measure pressure-pain threshold. Changes in sensory function associated with vertebral subluxation may produce changes in pressure-pain thresholds.
Rating: Established
Evidence: E, L

A pressure-pain threshold meter yields a measurement of when a patient feels a change from pressure to tenderness as the device produces mechanical irritation of deep somatic structures. Pressure-pain-threshold measurements produce acceptable levels of reliability.[62-66, 142-145] Algometry has been shown to be very useful in measuring changes in paraspinal tissue tenderness as the thresholds are symmetrical.[145] This renders the procedure applicable to chiropractic analysis.

CURRENT PERCEPTION THRESHOLD (CPT) TESTING

Sub-Recommendation

Current perception threshold devices may be used for the quantitative assessment of sensory nerve function. Alterations in sensory nerve function may be associated with vertebral subluxation.
Rating: Established
Evidence: E, L

The current perception threshold device is a variable voltage constant current sine wave stimulator proposed as a simple noninvasive and quantitative measure of peripheral nerve function.[67-71, 137-141] One type of current perception threshold instrument, the neurometer, has been shown to be appropriate for rapid screening for neural dysfunction.[69]

ELECTROENCEPHALOGRAPHY (EEG)

Sub-Recommendation

Electroencephalographic techniques including brain mapping and spectral analysis, may be used to assess the effects of vertebral subluxation and chiropractic adjustment associated with brain function.

Rating: Established
Evidence: E, L

Standard EEG and computerized EEG techniques, including spectral analysis and brain mapping, have been shown to change following chiropractic adjustments or manipulation.[72, 161, 204] Such procedures may be useful in evaluating possible effects of chiropractic care on brain function.

SOMATOSENSORY EVOKED POTENTIALS (SSEP)

Sub-Recommendation.

Somatosensory evoked potentials may be used for localizing neurological dysfunction associated with vertebral subluxations.
Rating: Established
Evidence: E, L

Somatosensory and dermatomal evoked potentials are used for localizing neurological abnormalities in the peripheral and central conducting pathways. These findings are useful as objective indicators of the level or levels of involvement.[73-86, 154] One study reported that improved nerve root function was observed in subjects who received a high-velocity chiropractic thrust; similar changes were not observed in controls.[73]

SKIN TEMPERATURE INSTRUMENTATION

Sub-Recommendation

Temperature reading devices employing thermocouples, infrared thermometry, or thermography (liquid crystal, telethermography, multiple IR detector, etc.) may be used to detect temperature changes in spinal and paraspinal tissues related to vertebral subluxation.
Rating: Established
Evidence: E, L

The measurement of paraspinal cutaneous thermal asymmetries and other measurements of anomalies have been shown to be a mode of sympathetic nervous system assessment, [88, 90, 91, 93-95, 97-103, 160] which may be used as one indicator of vertebral subluxation. Demonstrable changes in thermal patterns have been observed following chiropractic adjustment.[19, 92] Thermocouple instruments have been shown to demonstrate an acceptable level of reliability and clinical utility applicable to the assessment of vertebral subluxation related temperature changes.[87, 89, 96, 104] Normative data have been collected concerning the degree of thermal asymmetry in the human body in healthy subjects.[105] These values may serve as one standard in the assessment of sympathetic nerve function and the degree of asymmetry as a quantifiable indicator of possible dysfunction.[106]

SURFACE ELECTROMYOGRAPHY

Sub-Recommendation

Surface electrode electromyography, using hand-held electrodes, or affixed electrodes, may be used for recording changes in the electrical activity of muscles associated with vertebral subluxations.

Rating: Established
Evidence: E, L, C

Surface electromyographic techniques using both hand-held electrodes and affixed electrodes have demonstrated an acceptable level of reliability for general clinical usage.[107-112, 114-121, 129-136, 159] Other studies have demonstrated that significant changes in muscle electrical activity occur following adjustment or spinal manipulation.[111, 113, 126, 136] Protocols and normative data for paraspinal EMG scanning in chiropractic practice have been published.[122-125, 127-128] Surface EMG techniques may be used to assess changes in paraspinal muscle activity associated with vertebral subluxation and chiropractic adjustment.

MUSCLE STRENGTH TESTING

Sub-Recommendation

Muscle strength testing may be used to determine bilateral differences or other differences in patient resistance. These differences may be characterized by the experienced examiner based on various technologies. Manual, mechanized and computerized muscle testing may be used to determine changes in the strength and other characteristics of muscles. These changes may be a result of alterations of function at various levels of the neuromuscular system and/or any other system related to the patient. Such changes may be associated with vertebral subluxation.

Rating: Established
Evidence: E, L

Muscle testing as a means of evaluation and diagnosis of patients within chiropractic as well as other disciplines, is well documented.[146-153, 155-158, 163-177] Muscle testing techniques may be used to assess the effect of vertebral subluxation on various aspects of muscle strength. Research has shown manual muscle testing to be sufficiently reliable for clinical practice.[148, 149, 153, 156, 169, 170, 171, 175] Studies concerning manual muscle testing have also demonstrated electromyographic differences associated with various muscle weaknesses, and differences in somatosensory evoked potentials associated with weak versus strong muscles.[146, 147] Other studies have demonstrated the clinical utility and reliability of hand-held muscle strength testing devices.[151, 152, 157, 172]

QUESTIONNAIRES

Sub-Recommendation

Questionnaires may be used in the assessment of the performance of activities of daily living, pain perception, patient satisfaction, general health outcomes, patient perception outcomes, mental health outcomes, and overall quality of life, throughout a course of chiropractic care. Questionnaires provide important information, but should not be used as a substitute for physical indicators of the presence and character of vertebral subluxations.

Rating: Established

Evidence: E, L

There are a variety of questionnaires of demonstrated reliability and validity which may be used to document outcomes,[178-203] including pain and symptoms, although these are not necessary correlates of vertebral subluxation. However, correction of vertebral subluxation and reduction of the abnormal spinal and general functions associated with it may be accompanied by reduction or elimination of pain and symptoms. It must be emphasized that the clinical objective of chiropractic care is the correction of vertebral subluxations. No questionnaires exist which assess the presence or correction of vertebral subluxation. Therefore, it is inappropriate to employ questionnaires to determine the need for chiropractic care, but questionnaires are appropriate as one aspect of monitoring patient progress and the effectiveness of subluxation-based care.

References

1.   Vernon H. An assessment of the intra- and inter-reliability of the posturometer. J Manipulative Physiol Ther 1983; 6(2):57-60.

2.   Pearsall DJ, Reid JG, Hedden, DM. Comparison of three noninvasive methods for measuring scoliosis. Phys Ther 1992; 72(9):648-57.

3.   Adams A, Loper D, Willd S, et al. Intra- and inter-examiner reliability of plumb line posture analysis measurements using a 3-dimensional electrogoniometer. Res For 1988; 4(3):60-72.

4   Amendt LE, Ause-Ellias KL, Eybers JL, Wadsworth CT, Nielsen DH, Weinstein SL. Validity and reliability testing of the scoliometer. Phys Ther 1990; 70(2):108-17.

5.   Johnson GM: The correlation between surface measurement of head and neck posture and the anatomic position of the upper cervical vertebrae. Spine 1998; 23(8):921.

6.   Korovessis PG, Stamatakis MV. Prediction of scoliotic Cobb angle with the use of the scoliometer. Spine 1996; 21(14):1661-6.

7.   Grossman TV, Mazur JM, Cummings RJ. An evaluation of the Admas forward bend test and the scoliometer in a scoliosis school screening setting. J Pediatr Orthop 1995; 15(4):535-8.

8   Murrell GA, Coonrad RW, Moorman CT, 3d, Fitch RD. An assessment of the reliability of the scoliometer. Spine 1993; 18(6):709-12.

9.   Thomas E, Silman AJ, Papageorgiou AC, et al. Association between measures of spinal inability and low back pain: An analysis of new attenders in primary care. Spine 1998; 23(3):343-347.

10.   Chernuckha KU, Daffner RH, Reigel DH. Lumbar lordosis measurement. A new method versus Cobb technique. Spine 1998; 23(1):74-78.

11.   Haas M, Nyiendo J, Peterson C, et al. Interrater reliability of roentgenological evaluation of the lumbar spine in lateral bending. J Manipulative Physiol Ther 1990; 13(4):179-183.

12.   Owens E, Leach R. Changes in cervical curvature determined radiographically following chiropractic adjustment. Proceedings of the 1991 International Conference on Spinal Manipulation. April 12, 1991, Arlington, VA. Foundation for Chiropractic Education and Research.

13.   Plaugher G, Cremata E, Phillips R. A retrospective consecutive case analysis of pretreatment and comparative static radiological parameters following chiropractic adjustments. J Manipulative Physiol Ther, 1990; 13(9):498-503.

14.   Seemann DC. Bilateral weight differential and functional short leg: An analysis of pre and post data after reduction of an atlas subluxation. Chiropractic Research Journal 1993; 2(3):33-38.

15. Lawrence D. Lateralization of weight in the presence of structural short leg: A preliminary report. J Manipulative Physiol Ther 1984; 7(2):105-108.

16. Seeman D. A comparison of weight differential between a group that had a history of spinal problems or had been under care and a group that had neither a history of spinal problems or had been under care and a group that had neither a history of spinal problems nor been under care. Upper Cervical Monograph 1991; 5(2):17-19.

17. Herzog W, Nigg BM, Read LJ, Olsson E. Asymmetries in ground reaction force patterns in normal human gait. Med Sci Sports Exerc 21(1):110, 1989.

18. Vernon H, Grice A. The four-quadrant weight scale: A technical and procedural review. J Manipulative Physiol Ther 3:165, 1984.

19. Brand N, Gizoni C. Moiré contourography and infrared thermography: Changes resulting from chiropractic adjustments. J Manipulative Physiol Ther 1982; 5:113-116.

20. Laulund T, Sojbjerg J, Horlyck E. Moiré topography in school screening for structural scoliosis. ACTA Orthop Scand 1982; 53:765-768.

21. Ruggerone M, Austin J. Moiré topography in scoliosis: correlations with vertebral lateral curvature as determined by radiography. Phys Ther 1986; 66(7):1072-1077.

22. Spector B, Finando S, Fukuda F, Wilson S. An integrated video biofeedback/Moiré system for diagnosis and treatment: A preliminary report. J Manipulative Physiol Ther 3(4):220, 1980.

23. Spector B, Eilbert L, Fukuda F, Nystrom K. Development and application of spec-eil indices for quantitative analysis in moiré contourography. J Manipulative Physiol Ther 2(1): 16, 1979.

24. Van Wijk, M. Moiré Contourgraph—An accuracy analysis. Am Chiro 1981; 64-69.

25. Daruwalla J, Balasubramaniam P. Moiré topography in scoliosis—its accuracy in detecting the site and size of the curve. J Bone Joint Surg 1985; 67:211-213

26. Denton T, Randall F, Deinlein D. The use of instant moiré photographs to reduce exposure from sçoliosis radiographs. Spine 1992; 17(5):509-512.

27. East A, Kwan W. The application and validity of moiré topography in the screening of scoliosis. Eur J Chiro 1985; 33(2):108-130.

28. Eilbert L, Spector B. The moiré contourographic analysis controversy: a question of validity in present-day clinical practice. J Manipulative Physiol Ther 1979; 2:85.

29. El-Sayyad M. Comparison of roentgenography and moiré topography for quantifying spinal curvature. Phys Ther 1986; 66(7):1078-1082.

30. Sahlstrand T. The clinical value of moiré topography in the management of scoliosis. Spine 1986; 11:409-417.

31. Spector B, Finando S, Fukuda F, et al. An integrated video biofeedback/moiré system for diagnosis and treatment: a preliminary report. J Manipulative Physiol Ther 1980; 3(4):220-224.

32. Spector B, Fukuda F, Krammer L, et al. A preliminary integrated video biofeedback/moiré system. Am Chiro 1981; 14, 19.

33. Tibbles A, Belanger M, Grinder L, et al. Moiré topography in scoliosis screening: a study of the precision of the method. Proc of the Int'l Conf on Spinal Manip 1991; 43-44.

34. Stude D, Goertz C, Gallinger M. Inter- and intra-examiner reliability of a single, digital inclinometric range of motion measurement technique in the assessment of lumbar range of motion. J Manipulative Physiol Ther 1994; 17(2):83-87.

35. Lea, RD, Gerhardt JJ. Current Concepts Review: Range-of-Motion Measurements. J Bone Joint Surg, Vol 77-A(5):784-798, 1995.

36. Gerhardt, JJ, Rippstein JR: Measuring and Recording of Joint Motion. Instrumentation and Techniques. Toronto, Hogrefe and Huber, 1990.

37. Gerhardt, JJ. Documentation of Joint Motion. Revised ed. 4. Portland, Oregon, Isomed, 1994.

38. Petherick M, Rheault W, Kimble S, Lechner C, Senear V. Concurrent validity and intertester reliability of universal and fluid-based goniometers for active elbow range of motion. Phys Ther 58:996-969, 1988.

39. Asmussen E, Heeboll-Nielsen K. Posture, mobility and strength of the back in boys, 7 to 16 years old. ACTA Orthop Scand, 28: 174-189, 1959.

40. Keeley J, Mayer TG, Cox R, Gatchel RJ, Smith J, Mooney V. Quantification of lumbar function. Part 5: Reliability of range-of-motion measures in the sagittal plane and an in vivo torso rotation measurement technique. Spine, 11:31-35, 1986.

41. Loebl WY. Measurement of spinal posture and range of spinal movement. Ann Phys Med, 9:103-110, 1967.

42. Mayer TG. Rehabilitation of the patient with spinal pain. Orthop. Clin. North America, 14:623-637, 1983.

43. Mayer TG, Tencer AE, Kristoferson S, Mooney V. Use of noninvasive techniques for quantification of spinal range-of-motion in normal subjects and chronic low-back dysfunction patients. Spine, 9:588-595, 1984.

44. Portek L, Pearcy MJ, Reader GP, Mowat AG. Correlation between radiographic and clinical measurement of lumbar spine movement. British J Rheumatol., 22:197-205, 1983.

45. Reynolds PM. Measurement of spinal mobility: a comparison of three methods. Rheumat. and Rehab., 14:180-185, 1975.

46. Schober, VP. Lendenwirbelsaule und Kreuzschmerzen. Munchener med. Wochenschr., 84:336-338, 1937.

47. Tichauer, ER, Miller M, Nathan IM. Lordosimetry: a new technique for the measurement of postural response to materials handling. Am Indust Hyg Assn J, 34:1-12, 1973.

48. Troup JD, Hood CA, Chapman AE. Measurements of the sagittal mobility of the lumbar spine and hips. Ann Phys Med, 9:308-321, 1968.

49. Twomey LT, Taylor JR. Sagittal movements of the human lumbar vertebral column: a quantitative study of the role of the posterior vertebral elements. Arch Phys Med and Rehab, 64:322-325, 1983.

50. Kao MJ, Liao WS, Chen CY, Lai CL, Lien IN. Validity and reliability of measurement in the range of neck motion. Read at the Fifth General Assembly of the Asian Confederation for Physical Therapy, Taipei, Taiwan, Sept. 22, 1993.

51. Mayer TG, Tencer AF, Kristoferson S, Mooney V. Use of noninvasive techniques for quantification of spinal range-of-motion in normal subjects and chronic low-back dysfunction patients. Spine, 9:588-595, 1984.

52. Ebrall P. An estimation of the clinical error for the Metrecom computer-assisted goniometer. Chiropractic Technique 5 (1):1, 1993.

53. Ebrall P, Alevaki H, Cust S, Roberts N. An estimation of the measurement error of the Metrecom for computation of sagittal spinal angles. Chiropractic Technique 5 (3):104, 1993.

54. Chiarello C, Savidge R. Interrator reliability of the Cybex EDI-320 and fluid goniometer in normals and patients with low back pain. Archives of Physical Medicine and Rehabilitation 74: 32, 1993.

55. Dotson, LR, Luithens CA. A Comparison Between a Standard Manual Goniometer and the Metrecom Skeletal Analysis System. Presented at the South Florida Physical Therapy Association Meeting, North Miami Beach, FL, 1988.

56. Mior S, Clements D. A Comparison of X-Ray and Electrogoniometric Derived Cobb Angles: A Feasibility Study. Proc of the Int'l Conf on Spinal Manip 1992; 115.

57. Gill K, Krag MH, Johnson GB, Haugh LD, Pope MH. Repeatability of four clinical methods for assessment of lumbar spinal motion. Spine, 13:50-53, 1988.

58. American Medical Association: Guides to the Evaluation of Permanent Impairment. Ed. 4. Chicago, American Medical Association, 1993.

59. Ebrall P. An estimation of the clinical error for the Metrecom computer-assisted goniometer. Chiropractic Technique 1993; 5(1):1-4.

60. Waddell G, Somerville D, Henderson I, Newton M. Objective clinical evaluation of physical impairment in chronic low back pain. Spine, 17:617-628, 1992.

61. Gerhardt JJ. Measurements of ranges of motion and strength in evaluation of impairment. J Disabil 3:121-141, 1993.

62. Wallace H, Jahner S, Buckle K, Desai N. Correlation of the algometer neck disability index visual analog scale and the cervical spine curve in neck pain patients. J Manipulative Physiol Ther 17(4):292, 1994.

63. Fischer A. Application of pressure algometry in manual medicine. Manual Medicine 5 (4):145, 1990.

64. Reeves J, Jaeger B, Graff-Radford S. Reliability of the pressure algometer as a measure of myofascial trigger point sensitivity. Pain 24:313, 1986.

65. Fisher, AA. Pressure Algometry Over Normal Muscles: Standard Values, Validity and Reproducibility of Pressure Threshold. Pain 1989; 1:115-126.

66. Vernon H, Gitelman R. Pressure Algometry and Tissue Compliance Measures in the Treatment of Chronic Headache by Spinal Manipulation: A Single Case/Single Treatment Report. J Can Chiro Assoc 1990; 34(3):141-144.

67. Hill RS, Lawrence A. Current perception threshold and evaluating foot pain. Two case presentations. J Am Podiatr Med Assoc 81 (3):150, 1991.

68. Katims JJ, Rouvelas P, Sadler BT, Weseley SA. Current perception threshold. Reproducibility and comparison with nerve conduction in evaluation of carpal tunnel syndrome. ASAIO Trans 35(3):280, 1989.

69. Pitei DL, Watkins PJ, Stevens MJ, Edmonds ME. The value of the neurometer in assessing diabetic neuropathy by measurement of the current perception threshold. Diabet Med 11(9):872, 1994.

70. Katims JJ, Patil AS, Rendell M, et al. Current perception threshold screening for carpal tunnel syndrome. Archives of Environmental Health 46(4):207, 1991.

71. Vernon H, Aker P, Buns S, et al. Pressure pain threshold evaluation of the effect of a spinal manipulation in the treatment of chronic neck pain. J Manipulative Physiol Ther 13(1):13, 1990.

72. Hospers L. EEG and CEEG studies before and after upper cervical or SOT category II adjustment in children after head trauma in epilepsy and in "hyperactivity." Proceedings of the National Conference on Chiropractic and Pediatrics. November of 1992, 84-139.

73. Capria MP. Somatosensory neurological evaluation of chiropractic manipulation. Chiropractic: J Chiro Research and Clinical Investigation 6(3):56, 1990.

74. Collins K, Pfleger B. The neurophysiological evaluation of the subluxation complex: Documenting the neurological component with somatosensory evoked potentials. Chiropractic Research Journal 3(1):40, 1994.

75. Glick D, Lee F, Grostic J. Documenting the efficacy of chiropractic care utilizing somatosensory evoked potential testing. Proc of the Int'l Conf on Spinal Manip 1993, 82.

76. Grostic JD, Glick DM, Burke E, Sheres B. Chiropractic adjustment reversal of neurological insult: A Preliminary Report. Proc of the Int'l Conf on Spinal Manip 1992.

77. Collins KF, Pfleger B. The neurophysiological evaluation of the subluxation complex: Documenting the neurological component with somatosensory evoked potentials. Chiropractic Research Journal, 1994; 3(1):40-48.

78. Collins KF, Pfleger B. Significance of functional leg length inequality upon somatosensory evoked potential findings. Eleventh Annual Upper Cervical Spine Conference, Life College, 1994.

79. Grostic JD. Somatosensory evoked potentials in chiropractic research. Today's Chiropr, 56-58, 90.

80. Bamford C, Graeme K. Percutaneous S1 root somatosensory evoked potential. Electromyogr Clin Neurophysiol 1995; 35:181-186.

81. Chistyakov A, Soustiel J, Hafner H, et al. Motor and somatosensory conduction in cervical myelopathy and radiculopathy. Spine 1995; 20(19):2135-3140.

82. Glick D. Characterization of neurological insult in the low back utilizing somatosensory evoked potential studies. Proc of the Int'l Conf on Spinal Manip 1994; 17.

83. Kai Y, Owen J, Allen B, et al. Relationship between evoked potentials and clinical status in spinal cord ischemia. Spine 1994; 19(10):1162-1168.

84. Leppanen R, Maguire J, Wallace S, et al. Intraoperative lower extremity reflex muscle activity as an adjunct to conventional somatosensory-evoked potentials and descending neurogenic monitoring in idiopathic scoliosis. Spine 1995; 20(17):1872-1877.

85. Swenson R. Dermatomal somatosensory evoked potentials: A review of the literature. Journal of the Neuromusculoskeletal System 1994; 2(2):45-51.

86. Zhu Y, Hsieh C, Haldeman S, et al. Paraspinal muscle somatosensory evoked potentials in low back pain patients with muscle spasm: A quantitative study of the effect of spinal manipulation. Proc of the Int'l Conf on Spinal Manip 1994; 16.

87. Wallace H, Wallace J, Resh R. Advances in paraspinal thermographic analysis. Chiropractic Research Journal 2(3):39, 1993.

88. Abernathy M, Uematsu S. Medical Thermology. American Academy of Thermology, Georgetown University Medical Center, Washington, D.C.

89. Diakow, PRP. The status of thermography as a diagnostic tool. J Manipulative Physiol Ther 1990; 13(2):121.

90. Stewart MS, Riffle DW, Boone WR. Computer-aided pattern analysis of temperature differential. J Manipulative Physiol Ther. 1989; 12(5):345.352.

91. Hart J. Skin temperature patterns of the posterior neck used in chiropractic analysis- a case study. Chiropractic 1991; 7(2):46-48.

92. Hilliard K. Thermographic assessment of a toggle recoil adjusting treatment program. Proc of the Int'l Conf on Spinal Manip 1992; 117-118.

93. Erball P, Iggo A, Hobson P, et al. Preliminary report: The thermal characteristics of spinal levels identified as having different temperature by contact thermocouple measurement (Nervo Scope). Chiro J Aust 1994;24(4):139.

94. Kobrossi T. L5 and S1 nerve fiber irritation demonstrated by liquid crystal thermography-a case report. JCCA 1985; 29:199-202.

95. Schram S, Hosek R, Owens E. Computerized paraspinal skin surface temperature scanning: A technical report. J Manipulative Physiol Ther 1982; 5(3):117-121.

96. Pierce W, Stillwagon G. Charting and interpreting skin temperature differential patterns. Digest of Chiro Econ 1970; 12(5):37-9.

97. Fitzgerald P. Skin temperature patterns of the posterior neck used in chiropractic analysis. Chiropractic 1992; 8(1):1.

98. Hart J. Skin temperature patterns of the posterior neck used in chiropractic analysis. Chiropractic 1991; 7(2):46-48.

99. BenEliyahu DJ. Thermographic imaging of pathoneurophysiology due to cervical disc herniation. J Manipulative Physiol Ther 1989; 12:482-490.

100. Meeker W, Gahlinger P. Neuromuscular thermography: A valuable diagnostic tool? J Manipulative Physiol Ther 1986; 9:257-266.

101. Plaugher G. Skin temperature assessment for neuromuscular abnormalities of the spinal column: A review. Proc 6th Annual Conf on Research and Education, 1991.

102. Stillwagon G, Dalesio D. Chiropractic thermography. ICA Intl Rev Chiro 8-17, 1992.

103. Chafetz N, Wexler CE, Kaiser JA. Neuromuscular thermography of the lumbar spine with CT correlation. Spine 1988; 13:922-925.

104. Plaugher G, Lopes M, Melch P, et al. The inter- and intraexaminer reliability of a paraspinal skin temperature differential instrument. J Manipulative Physiol Ther 1991; 14(6):361-367.

105. Uematsu S. Symmetry of skin temperature comparing one side of the body to the other. Department of Neurosurgery, Johns Hopkins University School of Medicine, Baltimore, MD.

106. Uematsu S. Thermographic imaging of cutaneous sensory segment in patients with peripheral nerve injury. J Neurosurg 1985; 62:716-720.

107. Komi P, Buskirk E. Reproducibility of electromyographic measurements with inserted wire electrodes and surface electrodes. Electromyography 1970; 10:357.

108. Marcarian D. Factors influencing the SEMG's potential for continued future use. Transactions of the Consortium for Chiropractic Research 1993; 8:51-52.

109. Meyer J. The current status on validity of thoracolumbar paraspinal scanning EMG as a diagnostic test: A literature review. Transactions of the Consortium for Chiropractic Research 1993; 8:21-47.

110. Meyer J. The validity of thoracolumbar paraspinal scanning EMG as a diagnostic test: An examination of the current literature. J Manipulative Physiol Ther 1994; 17(8):539-551.

111. Myerowitz M. Scanning paraspinal Surface EMG: A method for corroborating post-treatment spinal and related neuromusculoskeletal symptom improvement. Journal of Occupational Rehabilitation 1994; 4(3):171-179.

112. Papakyriakou M, Triano J. Effects of filtering on the evaluation of surface EMG signals. Proc of the Int'l Conf on Spinal Manip 1993; 84.

113. Shambaugh P. Changes in electrical activity in muscles resulting from chiropractic adjustment: A Pilot Study. J Manipulative Physiol Ther 1987; 10(6):300-304.

114. Spector B. Surface electromyography as a model for the development of standardized procedures and reliability testing. J Manipulative Physiol Ther 1979; 2:214-222.

115. Triano J. Surface electrode EMG/lumbar spine: static paraspinal EMG scanning-clinical utility and validity issues. Transactions of the Consortium for Chiropractic Research 1993; 8:53-58.

116. Triano J. The validity of thoracolumbar paraspinal scanning EMG as a diagnostic test: examination of the current literature. J Manipulative Physiol Ther 1995; 18(7):482-483.

117. Ahern D, Follick M, Council J, et al. Reliability of lumbar paravertebral EMG assessment in chronic low back pain. Arch Phys Med Rehab 1986; 67:762.

118. Gentempo P, Kent C. Establishing medical necessity for paraspinal EMG scanning. Chiropractic: J Chiro Research and Clinical Investigation 1990; 3(1):22.

119. Gentempo P. Evaluating soft tissue injuries with electromyography-case studies. Today's Chiro 1988; 83.

120. Kent C, Fitzsimons W. Admissibility of electromyographic findings in personal injury cases, Digest Chiro Econ 1988; 30(5):43-46.

121. Kent C, Gentempo P. Medical evidence of soft tissue injury: legal aspects of paraspinal EMG findings. Am Chiro 1990; 12(12):10-15.

122. Kent C, Gentempo P. Protocol and normative data for paraspinal EMG scanning in chiropractic practice. Chiropractic: J Chiro Research and Clinical Investigation 1990; 6(3):64.

123. Kent C, Hyde R. Potential applications for electromyography in chiropractic practice. Digest Chiro Econ 1987; 30(2):20-25.

124. Kent C. Surface electrode EMG/lumbar spine. Transactions of the Consortium for Chiropractic Research 1993; 8:48.

125. Thompson D, Biederman H. Electromyographic power spectrum analysis of the paraspinal muscles. Spine 1993; 18(15):2310-2313.

126. Kent C. Surface electromyography in the assessment of changes in paraspinal muscle activity associated with vertebral subluxation: A review. Journal of Vertebral Subluxation Research. 1997; 1(3):15-22.

127. Miller EB, Redmond PD. Changes in digital skin temperature, surface electromyography, and electrodermal activity in subjects receiving network spinal analysis care. Journal of Vertebral Subluxation Research. 1998; 2(2):14-21.

128. Kent C, Gentempo P. Normative data for paraspinal surface electromyographic scanning using a 25-500 Hz band pass. Journal of Vertebral Subluxation Research, 1996; 1(1):43.

129. Giroux B, Lamontagne M. Comparisons between surface electrodes and intramuscular wire electrodes in isometric and dynamic conditions. Electromyogr Clin Neurophysiol 1990; 30:397.

130. Andersson G, Johnson B, Ortengren R. Myoelectric activity in individual lumbar erector spinal muscles in sitting. A study with surface and wire electrodes. Sc and J Rehab Med 1974; Suppl; 3:91.

131. Thompson J, Erikson R, Offord K. EMG muscle scanning: stability of hand-held electrodes. Biofeedback Self Requl 1989; 14(1):55.

132. Cram JR, Lloyd J, Cahn TS. The reliability of EMG muscle scanning. Int J Psychosomatics 1994; 41:41.

133. Boline P, Haas M, Meyer J, et al. Interexaminer reliability of eight evaluative dimensions of lumbar segmental abnormality: Part II. J Manipulative Physiol Ther 1993; 16(6):363-374.

134. Cram JR. Letter to the editor regarding interexaminer reliability of eight evaluative dimensions of lumbar segmental abnormality: Part II J Manipulative Physiol Ther 1994; 17(4):263.

135. Kent C, Gentempo P. Letter to the editor regarding Interexaminer reliability of eight evaluative dimensions of lumbar segmental abnormality: Part II J Manipulative Physiol Ther 1994; 17(7):495.

136. Ellestad S, Nagel R, Boesler D, et al. Electromyographic and skin resistance responses to osteopathic manipulative treatment for low-back pain. JAOA 1988; 88(8):991.

137. Katims JJ, Naviasky EH, Rendell MS, Ng LK, Bleecker ML. Constant current sine wave transcutaneous nerve stimulation for the evaluation of peripheral neuropathy. Arch Phys Med Rehabil. 1987; 68(4):210-3.

138. Evans ER, Rendell MS, Bartek JP, Bamisedun O, Connor S, Giitter M. Current perception thresholds in ageing. Age Ageing. 1992; 21(4):273-9.

139. Weseley SA, Sadler B, Katims JJ. Current perception: preferred test for evaluation of peripheral nerve integrity. ASAIO Trans. 1988; 34(3):188-93.

140. Katims JJ, Naviasky EH, Ng LK, Rendell M, Bleecker ML. New screening device for assessment of peripheral neuropathy. J Occup Med. 1986; 28(12):1219-21.

141. Masson EA, Beves A, Fernando D, et al. Current perception threshold: A new quick and reproducible method for the assessment of peripheral neuropathy in diabetes mellitus. Diabetologia 1989; 32:724-728.

142. Vatine JJ, Shapira SC, Magora F, Adler D, Magora A. Electronic pressure algometry of deep pain in healthy volunteers. Arch Phys Med Rehabil. 1993; 74(5):526-30.

143. Sandrini G, Antonaci F, Pucci E, Bono G, Nappi G. Comparative study with EMG, pressure algometry and manual palpation in tension-type headache and migraine. Cephalalgia. 1994; 14(6):451-7; discusson 394-5.

144. Kosek E, Ekholm J, Nordemar R. A comparison of pressure pain thresholds in different tissues and body regions. Long-term reliability of pressure algometry in healthy volunteers. Scand J Rehabil Med. 1993; 25(3):117-24.

145. Hogeweg JA, Langereis MJ, Bernards AT, Faber JA, Helders PJ. Algometry. Measuring pain threshold, method and characteristics in healthy subjects. Scand J Rehabil Med. 1992; 24(2):99-103.

146. Teisman G, Ferentz A, Zenhausern R, Tefera T, Zemoov A. Electromyographic effects of fatigue and task repetition on the validity of strong and weak muscle estimates in applied kinesiology muscle testing procedures: Perceptual and Motor Skills. 1995; 80:963-977.

147. Teisman G, Schambaugh P, Ferentz A. Somatosensory evoked potential changes during muscle testing. Intern J Neuroscience. 1989; 45:143-151.

148. Perot G, Meldener R, Goubol F. Objective measurement of proprioceptive technique consequences on muscular maximal voluntary contraction during manual muscle testing. Agressologic (French). 1991; 32(10):471-474.

149. Lawson A, Calderon I. Interexaminer reliability of applied kinesiology manual muscle testing. Perceptual and Motor Skills. 1997; 84:539-546.

150. Bender WL, Kaplan CM. The effectiveness of isometric testing as diagnostic aid: A hospital study. Journal of the Association for Physical and Mental Rehabilitation. 1962; 16:137-139.

151. Bohannan RW. Hand-held dynamometry: stability of music strength over multiple measurements. Clin Biomech 1986; 2:74.

152. Byl NN, Richards S, Asturias J. Intrarater and interrater reliability of strength measurements of the biceps and deltoid using a hand held dynamometer. J Orthop Sports Phys Ther 1988; 9:399.

153. Frese E, Brown M, Norton B. Clinical reliability of manual muscle testing. Middle trapezius and gluteus medius muscles. Phys Ther 1987; 67(7):1072-1076.

154. Glick DM, Lee F. Differential diagnostic somatosensory evoked potentials. Chiropractic Research Journal 1991; 2(2):38.

155. Hsieh J, Gilbertson K. Reliability of mean power frequency and median power frequency in bilateral upper trapezius isometric work. Proc of the Int'l Conf on Spinal Manip 1993; 21.

156. Saraniti AJ, Gleim GW, Melvin M, et al. The relationship between subjective and objective measurements of strength. J Orthop Sports Phys Ther 1980; 2:15.

157. Silverman JL, Rodriquez AA, Agre JC. Reliability of hand-held dynanometer in neck strength testing. Arch Phys Med Rehab 1989; 70(Suppl):94.

158. Hseih J, Phillips R. Reliability of manual muscle testing with a computerized dynamometer. J Manipulative Physiol Ther 1990; 13(2):72.

159. Thabe J. Electromyography as a tool to document diagnostic findings and therapeutic results associated with somatic dysfunction in the upper cervical spinal joints and sacro-iliac joints. Manual Med 1986; 2:53-58.

160. Wexler C, Small R. Thermographic demonstration of a sensory nerve deficit: A case report. Journal of Neurological and Orthopaedic Surgery 1981; 3(1).

161. Dretakis E, Paraskevaidis C, Zarkadoulas V, Christodoulou N. Electroencephalographic study of schoolchildren with adolescent idiopathic scoliosis. Spine. 1988; 13:143-5.

162. Carrick FR. Changes in brain function after manipulation of the cervical spine. J Manipulative Physiol Ther, 1997; 8:529-545.

163. Bonci A, Ratliff C. Strength modulation of the biceps brachii muscles immediately following a single manipulation of the C4/5 intervertebral motor unit in healthy subjects: preliminary report. Am J Chiro Med 1990; 3(1):14-18.

164. Brodie D, Callaghan M, Green A. Ergotest 2000 - a new device for muscle testing and rehabilitation Physiotherapy 1990; 76(7):412-415.

165. Bussieres A, Mior S, Frazer M, et al. Cervical motion and muscle strength measurements: A comparative study of symptom free and neck pain subjects. Proc of the Int'l Conf on Spinal Manip 1994; 110-111.

166. Chapman, S. Isokinetics: muscle testing, interpretation and clinical applications. J Manipulative Physiol Ther 1995; 18(6):424-425.

167. Finucane S, Walker M, Rothstein J, et al. Reliability of isometric muscle testing of knee flexor and extensor muscles in patients with connective tissue disease. Phys Ther 1988; 68(3):338-343.

168. Grossi J. Effects of an applied kinesiology technique on quadriceps femoris muscle isometric strength. Phys Ther 1981; 61:1011-1016.

169. Haas M, Peterson D, Hoyer D, et al. Muscle testing response to provocative vertebral challenge and spinal manipulation: A randomized controlled trial of construct validity. J Manipulative Physiol Ther 1994; 17(3):141-148.

170. Hsieh C, Phillips R. Reliability of manual muscle testing with a computerized dynamometer. J Manipulative Physiol Ther 1990; 13(2):72-82.

171. Hyytiainen K, Salminen J, Suvitie T, et al. Reproducibility of nine tests to measure spinal mobility and trunk muscle strength. Scand J Rehabil Med 1991; 23:3-10.

172. Mannello D, Sanders G, Kavalin J. The ability of the Dynatron 2000 to detect effort level. J Manipulative Physiol Ther 1991; 13(2):122.

173. Newton M, Waddell G. Trunk strength testing with iso-machines: Part 1: Review of a decade of scientific evidence. Spine 1993; 18(7):801-811.

174. Vernon H, Aker P, Aramenko M, et al. The use of a modified sphygmomanometer dynamometer in isometric strength tests in the neck: Reliability and normative data. Proc of the Int'l Conf on Spinal Manip 1990; 170-173.

175. Vernon H, Aker P, Menko M, et al. Evaluation of neck muscle strength with a modified sphygmomanometer dynamometer: Reliability and Validity. J Manipulative Physiol Ther 1992; 15(6):343-349.

176. Vernon H. Sincerity of effort in neck muscle strength testing - An analogue study. Proc of the Int'l Conf on Spinal Manip 1992; 82-83.

177. Westers B. Factors influencing strength testing and exercise prescription. Physiotherapy 1982; 68(2):42-44.

178. McDowell J, Newell C. Measuring health: A guide to rating scales and questionnaires. 1st ed. New York: Oxford University Press, 1996.

179. Tennant A, Badley E. A confidence interval approach to investigating non-response bias and monitoring response to postal questionnaires. Journal of Epidemiology and Community Health 1991; 45:81-85.

180. Tennant A, Badley E. Investigating non-response bias in a survey of disablement in the community: implications for survey methodology. Journal of Epidemiology and Community Health 1991; 45:247-250.

181. Diener E, Suh E, Smith H, et al. National differences in reported subjective well-being: Why do they occur? Social Indicators Research 1995; 34:7-32.

182. Torrance G. Utility approach to measuring health-related quality of life. J Chron Dis 1987; 40(6):593-600.

183. Grant M, Ferrell B, Schmidt GM, et al. Measurement of quality of life in bone marrow transplantation survivors. Quality of Life Research 1992; 1:375-384.

184. Wilson I, Cleary P. Linking clinical variables with health-related quality of life. A conceptual model of patient outcome. JAMA1995; 273(1):59-65.

185. Kenney J. The consumer's views of health. Journal of Advanced Nursing 1992; 17(7):829-834.

186. Commentary. Choosing measures of health status for individuals in general populations. AJPH 1981; 71:620-625.

187. Kirshner B, Guyatt Gordon. A methodological framework for assessing health indices. J Chron Dis 1985; 38(1)27-36.

188. Pavot W, Diener E. The affective and cognitive context of self-reported measures of subjective well-being. Social Indicators Research 1993; 28:1-20.

189. Diener E. Assessing subjective well-being: progress and opportunities. Social Indicators Research 1994; 31:103-157.

190. Andersson G, Weinstein J. Introduction: health outcomes related to low back pain. Spine 1994; 19(18S):2026S-7S.

191. Bronfront G. An overview of short multi-dimensional health status outcomes instruments. Northwestern College of Chiropractic.

192. Cherkin DC. Patient satisfaction as an outcome measure. J Chiropracic Tech 1990; 2(3) 138.

193. Haas M, Jacobs G, Raphael R, et al. Responsiveness and applicability of two functional disability questionnaires in the chiropractic teaching clinic setting. Western State College and Cleveland College of Chiropractic.

194. Haas M, Nyiendo J. Diagnostic utility of the McGill Pain Questionnaire and the Oswestry Disability Questionnaire for classification of low back pain syndromes. J Manipulative Physiol Ther 1992; 15(22):90-98.

195. Hagino C, Papernick L. Test-retest reliability of the 'CMCC Low Back Status Questionnaire for Laypersons.' Proc of the Int'l Conf on Spinal Manip A/M 1993; 47.

196. Hains F, Waalen J, Mior S. Psychometric properties of the Neck Disability Index; final results. Proc of the Int'l Conf on Spinal Manip 1994; 8-9.

197. Hawk C, Wallace H, Dusio M. Development of a global well-being scale: A study of reliability, validity and responsiveness. Proc of the Int'l Conf on Spinal Manip 1994; 41-42.

198. Jaeschke R, Singer J, Guyatt G. A comparison of seven-point and visual analog scales: Data from a randomized trial. Controlled Clin Trials 11:43-51, 1990.

199. Lawlis G, Cuencas R, Selby D, et al. The development of the Dallas Pain Questionnaire: An assessment of the impact of spinal pain on behavior. Spine 1989; 14(5)511-516.

200. Love A, Leboeur C, Crisp T. Chiropractic chronic low back pain sufferers and self-report assessment methods. Part I. A reliability study of the visual analogue scale, the pain drawing and the McGill. J Manipulative Physiol Ther 1989; 12(1)21-25.

201. Nylendo J, Haas M, Jones R. Using the SF-36D (General Health Questionnaire) in a pilot study of outcome assessment for low back chiropractic patients. Proc of the Int'l Conf on Spinal Manip FCER, Arlington, VA. 172, 1991.

202. Sawyer, C. Patient satisfaction as a chiropractic research outcome. Proc Int'l Conf on Spinal Manip. FCER, Arlington, VA. 163, 1991.

203. Blanks RHI, Schuster T, Dobson M. A retrospective assessment of Network Care using a survey of self-rated health, wellness and quality of life. Journal of Vertebral Subluxation Research, 1997; 1(4):15-31.

204. Holder JM. New technique introduced. EEG confirms results. ILAC Journal, May 1996: 10.

3 Radiographic and Other Imaging

RECOMMENDATION

Diagnostic imaging procedures may be utilized to characterize the biomechanical manisfestations of vertebral subluxation, and to determine the presence of conditions which affect the safety and appropriateness of chiropractic care.

Sub-Recommendation

Plain film radiography is indicated: to provide information concerning the structural integrity of the spine, skull and pelvis; the misalignment component of the vertebral subluxation; the foraminal alteration component of the vertebral subluxation; and the postural status of the spinal column. Imaging procedures, including post-adjustment radiography, should be performed only when clinically necessary. It is common for lines of mensuration to be drawn on radiographs to assess subluxation and alignment. These procedures may be done by hand, or the chiropractor may utilize computerized radiographic digitization procedures.

Rating: Established
Evidence: E, L

Commentary

In considering the use of imaging methods employing ionizing radiation as a component of patient assessment, the clinician should determine if the methods of subluxation correction, patient safety, and management require the use of such procedures. The patient should be asked about any conditions which may contraindicate certain imaging procedures.

Reliability studies of several systems of biomechanical analysis, including radiographic marking systems, have been published. Imaging is a necessary component of a number of different chiropractic analyses. The preponderance of evidence supports the reliability of these procedures when properly performed.[1-8, 12, 15-27, 29-32, 36-39, 42-61, 64-68, 70-79, 153]

Moreover, radiographic imaging has revealed statistically significant changes in the direction of atlas positioning following chiropractic adjustment(s).[14, 28, 33-35, 146-148] The effect of chiropractic care on lateral curvature of the cervical spine has been investigated, with significant changes in the cervical curve noted in patients receiving chiropractic care.[9, 62, 63, 69, 149-152, 156-158]

Sub-Recommendation

Imaging procedures employing ionizing radiation should be performed consistent with the principles of obtaining films of high quality with minimal

radiation. This may include the use of gonad shielding, compensating filters, and appropriate film-screen combinations.
Rating: Established
Evidence: E, L

A number of dosimetry studies using supplemental filtration and single-speed screens have revealed that in the case of 14 x 36 inch AP full-spine radiographs, the radiation levels were less than sectional films of like-sized subjects. Shielding of radiosensitive structures may be used when it does not obliterate structures of clinical interest. Such shielding results in a reduction of radiation exposure.[10, 11, 13, 160]

Conclusion

The judicious use of spinographic techniques can be valuable in characterizing aspects of the biomechanical manifestations of vertebral subluxation.[146, 154, 155, 187-193] The use of post-adjustment radiographs may also assist the chiropractor in determining effects of chiropractic adjustments on the spine when other less hazardous examination techniques cannot reveal the desired information.

VIDEOFLUOROSCOPY

Sub-Recommendation

Videofluoroscopy may be employed to provide motion views of the spine when abnormal motion patterns are clinically suspected. Videofluoroscopy may be valuable in detecting and characterizing spinal kinesiopathology associated with vertebral subluxation.
Rating: Established
Evidence: E, L

Commentary

A videofluoroscopic system consists of an x-ray generator capable of operating at low (1/4 to 5) milliamperage settings, an x-ray tube assembly, an image intensifier tube, a television camera, a VCR, and a monitor. The heart of the system is the image intensifier tube. This tube permits imaging at very low radiation levels. It is used instead of intensifying screens and film as a image receptor.

The role of videofluoroscopy in the evaluation of abnormalities of spinal motion has been discussed in textbooks, medical journals, and chiropractic publications.[19, 20, 23, 80-83, 140, 145, 163, 164, 168-170, 172-179, 186, 220] Studies have appeared in the literature comparing the diagnostic yield of fluoroscopic studies versus plain films, as well as reporting abnormalities detected by fluoroscopy which could not be assessed using plain films.[161, 165-167, 171, 180, 183-185]

Reliability has been addressed in a number of studies.[162, 181, 182, 214] Additionally, in a study evaluating the interexaminer reliability of fluoroscopic detection of fixation in the mid-cervical spine, two examiners reviewed 50 videotapes of fluoroscopic examinations of the cervical spine. The examiners achieved 84 percent agreement for the presence of fixation, 96 percent agreement for the absence of fixation, and 93 percent total agreement. The Kappa value was .80 (p<.001). The authors concluded, "The current data indicate that VF determination of fixation in the cervical spine is a reliable procedure." [181, 214]

Conclusion

Observational and case studies support the use of videofluoroscopy to evaluate vertebral motion when this information cannot be obtained by other means.

Sub-Recommendation

Magnetic Resonance Imaging (MRI)

MR imaging may be employed to assess suspected neoplastic, infectious and degenerative conditions of the spine and related tissues as well as the stages of subluxation degeneration. Its use is generally restricted to instances where the desired information cannot be obtained by less costly procedures.

Rating: Established
Evidence: E, L

Commentary

Magnetic resonance imaging enables clinicians to obtain clear images of the human body without ionizing radiation.

Literature supports the use of MR imaging for the detection and characterization of numerous manifestations associated with subluxation degeneration.[84-107, 141-143, 194-198, 212] These studies cover a spectrum of phenomena, including:

1. Osseous malalignment
2. Intervertebral disc desiccation and degeneration
3. Osteophytosis
4. Corrugation/hypertrophy of the ligamentum flava
5. Spinal canal stenosis
6. Foraminal stenosis
7. Disc herniation and disc bulging
8. Facet asymmetry
9. Facet degeneration
10. Altered cerebrospinal fluid dynamics
11. Cord compression
12. Gliosis and myelomalacia
13. Spinal cord atrophy

Conclusion

MRI may be employed to disclose manifestations of vertebral subluxation when this information cannot be obtained by more cost-effective means. MRI is also appropriate for evaluating patients with clinical evidence of conditions which may affect the safety and appropriateness of chiropractic procedures.

Sub-Recommendation

Computed Tomography (CT)

CT imaging may be employed to assess osseous and soft tissue pathology in the spine and contiguous tissues. Its use is generally restricted to instances where the desired information cannot be obtained by less costly procedures.
Rating: Established
Evidence: E, L

Commentary

Computed tomography (also referred to as CT or CAT scanning) is an imaging technique which produces axial (cross sectional) images of body structures using x-radiation. Computer reconstruction methods may be used to depict other planes.

Manifestations of subluxation degeneration which may be demonstrated by CT scanning include disc lesions, spinal canal stenosis due to infolding of the ligamentum flava, osteophytosis, and bony sclerosis.[108-139, 144, 199-201, 210, 211, 213, 220] In addition, CT may be used to evaluate developmental variance and pathologies which could affect the chiropractic management of a case.

Conclusion

CT may be employed to disclose manifestations of vertebral subluxation when this information cannot be obtained by more cost-effective means. CT is also appropriate for evaluating patients with clinical evidence of conditions which may affect the safety and appropriateness of chiropractic procedures, particularly fractures, degenerative changes, and osseous pathology.

Sub-Recommendation

Spinal Ultrasonography

Spinal ultrasonography may be used to evaluate the size of the spinal canal, and to detect pathology in the soft tissues surrounding the spine. Its applications in the assessment of the facet inflammation and nerve root inflammation remain investigational at this time.
Ratings: Established for determining spinal canal size.
Investigational for facet and nerve root inflammation.
Evidence: E, L

Commentary

Sonographic imaging is a technique which utilizes echoes from ultrasonic waves to produce an image on a cathode ray tube.

Sonographic techniques have been employed to measure the lumbar canal, as well as determining focal stenosis and disc disease.[202-209, 221, 222]

A small study compared sonographic results in patients with back pain previously examined by MRI, x-ray and standard orthopedic examination. The study concluded that the correlation with MRI, x-ray, orthopedic and neurologic examination was approximately 90 percent.[207]

Conclusion

The low cost, availability, ease of application, and noninvasive nature of sonographic imaging make it an attractive addition to the chiropractor's armamentarium. Furthermore, it has the potential to image various components of the vertebral subluxation. However, caution must be exercised in evaluating the claims of promoters of sonographic equipment, particularly those relating to the assessment of nerve root inflammation or facet joint disease. Further research toward the establishment of chiropractic protocols should be undertaken to explore the clinical utility of spinal sonography in chiropractic practice.

Sub-Recommendation

Radioisotope Scanning (Nuclear Medicine Studies)

Radioisotope scans performed by qualified medical personnel may be used by a chiropractor to determine the extent and distribution of pathological processes which may affect the safety and appropriateness of chiropractic care when this information cannot be obtained by less invasive means.
Rating: Established
Evidence: E, L

Commentary

In this procedure, bone-seeking radioisotopes are injected, and an image is produced demonstrating the degree of uptake of the radioisotopes. The examination is sensitive to regional changes in osseous metabolism, but is not specific. Abnormal bone scans may be due to metastasis, infection, fracture, osteoblastic activity or other pathology.[215-219] No studies or case reports were found linking abnormal bone scans with vertebral subluxation. Bone scans may have limited value in determining the safety and appropriateness of chiropractic procedures.

Conclusion

Radioisotope scans have a limited role in chiropractic practice. Bone scans are a sensitive, but nonspecific indicator of abnormal metabolic activity in bone.

References

1. Rochester RP. Inter- and intra-examiner reliability of the upper cervical x-ray marking system: A third and expanded look. Chiropractic Research Journal 1994; 3(1):23-31.

2. Seemann DC. Observer reliability and objectivity using rotatory measurements on x-rays. Upper Cervical Monograph 1986; 4(1):1, 68.

3. Seemann DC. A reliability study using a positive nasium to establish laterality. Upper Cervical Monograph 1994; 5(4):7, 8.

4. Rochester RP, Owens EF. Patient placement error in rotation and its affect on the upper cervical measuring system. Chiropractic Research Journal 1996; 3(2):40-53.

5. Suh CH. The fundamentals of computer aided x-ray analysis of the spine. J Biomechanics 1974; 7:161-169.

6. Suh CH. Minimum error point search for spinal x-ray analysis. Chiropractic Research Journal 1988; 1(1):4-12.

7. Suh CH. Displacement analysis of the spine with use of x-rays. Chiropractic Research Journal 1988; 1(2):5-16.

8. Grostic JD. Some observations on computer-aided x-ray analysis. Internat Rev Chiropr, July-September 1979, pp. 38-41.

9. McAlpine JE. Subluxation induced cervical myelopathy: A pilot study. Chiropractic Research Journal 1991; 2(1):7-22.

10. Dickholtz M. Comments and concerns re x-ray radiation (A guide for upper cervical x-ray). The Upper Cervical Monograph 1989; 4(8):7-9.

11. Eriksen K. Reducing x-ray exposure. The Atlas 1996; 1(2):2, 3.

12. Eriksen K. Comparison between upper cervical x-ray listings and technique analyses utilizing a computerized database. Chiropractic Research Journal 1996; 3(2):13-24.

13. Eriksen K, Owens EF. Upper cervical post x-ray reduction and its relationship to symptomatic improvement and spinal stability. Chiropractic Research Journal 1997; 4(1):10-17.

14. Grostic J. Roentgenographic measurement of atlas laterality and rotation: A retrospective pre- and post-manipulation sudy. J Manipulative Physiol Ther 1982; 5(2)63.

15. Hadley L. Anatomical and roentgenographic studies of the spine. CC Thomas, IL, 1981.

16. Hass M, Nylendo J. Lumbar motion trends and correlation with low back pain. A roentgenographic evaluation of quantitative segmental motion in lateral bending. Proc 1991 World Chiro Congr Toronto, 1991.

17. Plaugher G, Cremata E, Phillips R. A retrospective consecutive case analysis of pre-treatment and comparative static radiological parameters following chiropractic adjustments. J Manipulative Physiol Ther 1990; 13(1)57.

18. El-Sayyad M. Comparison of roentgenography and moiré topography for quantifying spinal curvature. Phys Ther, 1986; 66(7):1078-1082.

19. Armstrong P, Wastic ML. Diagnostic Imaging, 2nd Ed. Blackwell Scientific Publications, Oxford, 1987.

20. Ball and Moore: Essential physics for radiographers, 2nd Ed. Blackwell Scientific Publications, St. Louis, Mo., 1987.

21. Hildebrandt RW. Chiropractic Spinography—A manual of technology and interpretation. Hilmark Publication, Des Plains, IL, 1977.

22. Kent C, Gentempo P. The documentary basis for diagnostic imaging procedures in the subluxation-based chiropractic practice. International Chiropractors Association, 1992.

23. Kent, C. Contemporary technologies for imaging the vertebral subluxation complex. ICA Review 1989; 45(4): 45-51.

24. Selman J. The fundamentals of x-ray and radiation physics, 7th Ed. CC Thomas Publ, 1986.

25. X-ray examinations (A guide to good practice). U.S. Dept. of Health, Education, and Welfare. USPHS, 1971.

26. Plaugher G, Hendricks A, Doble R, et al. The reliability of patient positioning for evaluating static radiologic parameters of the human pelvis. J Manipulative Physiol Ther 1993; 16(8):517-522.

27. Taylor, J. Full-spine radiography: A review of the literature. Transactions of the Consortium for Chiropractic Research 1992; 7:190-216.

28. Sherwood K, Brickner D, Jennings D. Postural changes after reduction of the atlantal-axial subluxation. Chiropractic Research Journal 1989; 96-100.

29. Haas M, Nyiendo J, Peterson C, et al. Interrater reliability of roentgenological evaluation of the lumbar spine in lateral bending. J Manipulative Physiol Ther 1990; 13(4)179-189.

30. Hon T, Smith R. Interrater reliability of roentgenological evaluation of the lumbar spine in lateral bending. J Manipulative Physiol Ther 1991; 14(2)158.

31. Lane, M. A radiographic study of the movement of the innominate with respect to the sacrum about the sacroiliac joint. Bull Eur Chiro Union 1976; 24(1)41-47.

32. Lantz, C. Interrater reliability of roentgenological evaluation of the lumbar spine in lateral bending. J Manipulative Physiol Ther 1991; 14(5)329-331.

33. McGregor M, Mior S, Shannon H, et al. The clinical usefulness of flexion-extension radiographs in the cervical spine. Topics in Clinical Chiropractic 1995; 2(3)19-28.

34. Mior S, Clements D. A comparison of x-ray and electrogoniometric derived Cobb angles: A feasibility study. Proc of the Int'l Conf on Spinal Manip 1992; 115.

35. Jirout, J. Roentgen studies of the cervical spine. Radiologic Clinic, Dept of Neuroradiology, Charles Univ Prague, Czechoslovakia. Gustav-Fischer-Verlag, Stuttgart, Germany (translated to English by author).

36. Dailey E, Buehler M. Plain Film Assessment of Spinal Stenosis: Method Comparison with Lumbar CT. J Manipulative Physiol Ther 1989; 12:192-199.

37. Zengel F, Davis B. Biomechanical analysis by chiropractic radiography: Part II. Effects of x-ray projectional distortion on apparent vertebral rotation. J Manipulative Physiol Ther 1988; 11(5): 380-389.

38. Zengel F, Davis B. Biomechanical analysis by chiropractic radiography: Part I. A simple method for determining x-ray projectional distortion. J Manipulative Physiol Ther 1988; 11(4): 273-280.

39. DeVilliers PD, Booysen EL. Fibrous spinal stenosis, a report of 850 myelograms with a water-soluble contrast medium. Clin Orthop 1976; 115:140-144.

40. Larsen JL. The lumbar spinal canal in children: II. The interpedicular distance and its relation to the sagittal diameter and transverse pedicular width. Eur J Radiol 1981; 1:312-321.

41. Eisenstein S. Measurement of the lumbar spinal canal in 2 racial groups. Clin Orthop 1976; 115:42-46.

42. Dailey EJ, Buehler MT. Plain film assessment of spinal stenosis: Method comparison with lumbar CT. J Manipulative Physiol Ther 1989; 3:192-199.

43. Burns S, Mior S, McGregor M, et al. Identifying errors in cervical spinal canal measurements. Proc of the World Chiro Congress, 1991.

44. Deboer K. Inter- and intra-examiner reliability of the upper cervical x-ray marking system. J Manipulative Physiol Ther 1985; 8(4): 285-286.

45. Grostic J, Marshall W. Accuracy of an upper cervical measuring system: A validity study. Proc of the Int'l Conf on Spinal Manip 1992; 146-147.

46. Jackson B, Barker W, Bentz J, et al. Inter- and intra-examiner reliability of the upper cervical x-ray marking system: a second look. J Manipulative Physiol Ther 1987; 10(4):157-163.

47. Jackson B. Reliability of the upper cervical x-ray marking system: A replication study. Chiropractic Research Journal 1998; 1(1):10-13.

48. Keating J. Interexaminer/intertechnique reliability in spinal subluxation assessment: a multifactorial approach. Am J Chiro Med 1989; 2(1):30.

49. Keating J. The precision and reliability of an upper cervical x-ray marking system: lessons from the literature. Chiropractic Research Journal 1988; 4:32-42.

50. Moroney S, Plaugher G, Cremata E, et al. An analysis of the accuracy of a biplanar radiographic algorithm: The simulated motions of a mathematical model and the calculated motions of a calibrated physical model. Proc of the Int'l Conf on Spinal Manip 1990; 99-101.

51. Owens E, Hosek R. Structure location errors in an upper cervical x-rays analysis. Chiropractic Research Journal 1988; 1(1): 13-20.

52. Owens E. Line drawing analyses of static cervical x-ray used in chiropractic. J Manipulative Physiol Ther 1992; 15(7): 442-449.

53. Owens E, Hoirris K. Cervical curvature assessment using digitized radiographic analysis. Chiropractic Research Journal 1990; 1(4):47-62.

54. Palmer J. Inter- and intra-examiner reliability of the upper cervical x-ray marking system. J Manipulative Physiol Ther 1985; 8(4):285.

55. Plaugher G, Hendricks A. The Inter- and intra-examiner reliability of the gonstead pelvic marking system. J Manipulative Physiol Ther 1991; 14(9):503-508.

56. Rochester, R. Inter and intra-examiner reliability of the upper cervical x-ray marking system: A third and expanded look. Chiropractic Research Journal; 3(1):23-31.

57. Sansone M, Wooley J, Grannis G. Inter- and intra-examiner reliability of upper cervical x-ray marking system. J Manipulative Physiol Ther 1986; 9(4):285.

58. Schram S, Hosek R. Error limitations in x-ray kinematics of the spine. J Manipulative Physiol Ther 1982; 5(1): 5-10.

59. Schram, S. Analysis of errors in x-ray measurements of cervical vertebrae. Proc of the Biomechanics Conf on the Spine 1980; 93-111.

60. Sigler D, Howe J. Inter- and intra-examiner reliability of the upper cervical x-ray marking system. J Manipulative Physiol Ther 1985; 8:75-80.

61. Sigler, D. Inter- and intraexaminer reliability of the upper cervical x-ray marking system: A second look. J Manipulative Physiol Ther 1988; 11(3):228-229.

62. Mears, D. Adjustment of subluxations as analyzed on lateral cervical x-rays. Digest Chiro Econ 1972; 14(6):14-15.

63. Mears, D. Analysis and adjustment of the occiput and cervical spine. Digest Chiro Econ 1970; 12(4):52-53.

64. Beekman C. Variability of scoliosis measurement from spinal roentgenograms. Phys Ther 1979; 59: 764-765.

65. Bellamy N, Newhook L, Rooney P. Perception—A problem in the grading of sacro-iliac joint radiographs. Scand J Rheumatol 1984; 13:13-120.

66. Carman D, Browne R, Birch J. Measurement of scoliosis and kyphosis radiographs. J Bone Joint Surg 1990; 72A(3):328-333.

67. Cockshott W, Park W. Observer variation in skeletal radiology. Skeletal Radiol 1983; 10:86-90.

68 Dailey E, Buehler M. Plain film assessment of spinal stenosis: Method comparison with lumbar CT. J Manipulative Physiol Ther 1989; 12(3):92-199.

69. Herring C. Static cervical x-ray analysis as utilized in Herring technique. Transactions of the Consortium for Chiropractic Research 1991; 121-139.

70. Herzog R. Imaging corner: The goal of spinal imaging. Spine 1994; 19(21):2486-2488.

71. Mannello D. Inter-rater agreement of basic technique radiographic analysis. Transactions of the Consortium for Chiropractic Research 1993; 8:158-159.

72. Mick, T. The use of functional radiographs in diagnosis: A literature review. Transactions of the Consortium for Chiropractic Research 1992; 7:108-167.

73. Morrissy R, Goldsmith G, Hall E. Measurement of the Cobb angle on radiographs of patients who have scoliosis. J Bone Joint Surg 1990; 72A(3):320-327.

74. Portek I, Pearcy M, Reader G, et al. Correlation between radiographic and clinical measurement of lumbar spine movement. BR J Rheumatol 1983; 22:197-205.

75. Rupert, R. Anatomical measures of standard chiropractic skeletal references (a preliminary report). Proc of the Biomechanics Conf on the Spine 1980; 11:83-92.

76. Taylor J, Clopton P, Bosch E, et al. Interpretation of abnormal lumbosacral spine radiographs: A test comparing students, clinicians, radiology residents, and radiologists in medicine and chiropractic. Spine 1995; 20(10):1147-1154.

77. Taylor J. Full-spine radiography: A review of the literature. Transactions of the Consortium for Chiropractic Research 1992; 7:190-216.

78. Thorkeldsen A, Breen A. Gray scale range and the marking of vertebral coordinates on digitized radiographic images. J Chiro 1994; 17(6):359-363.

79. Yamagata M, Inoue S, Moriya H, et al. Three-dimensional measurement of the scoliotic spine using biplanar radiographic method. J West Pac Orthop Assoc 1990; 27:95-100.

80. Wallace H, Pierce W, Wagon R. Cervical flexion and extension analysis using digitized videofluoroscopy. Chiropractic: J Chiro Research and Clinical Investigation 1992; 7(4)94-97.

81. Bushong SC. Radiologic science for technologists, 4th Ed. The C.V. Mosby Company, St. Louis, Mo. 1988; 1-621.

82. Kent C. The role of videofluoroscopy in chiropractic practice. ICA Review 1990; 46(1):41-45.

83. Mauer E. Biological effects of x-ray exposure. Am J Chiro Med 1988; 1(3):115-118.

84. Kent C, Holt F, Gentempo P. Subluxation Degeneration in the Lumbar Spine: Plain Film and MR Imaging Considerations. ICA Review 1991; 47(1):55-59.

85. Kent C, Gentempo P. Subluxation degeneration in the cervical spine: Plain film and MRI findings. ICA Review 1991; 47(4):47.

86. Kent C, Gentempo P. MR imaging of subluxation degeneration. Chiropractic Research Journal 1990; 1(4):39.

87. Bishop PB. Intervertebral disc magnetic resonance image: Correlation with gross morphology and biochemical composition. J Can Chiro Assoc 1993; 37:77-84.

88. Abdelwahab IF, Kenan S, Hermann G, Klein MJ, Lewis MJ, Lewis MM. Periosteal ganglia: CT amd MR imaging features. Radiology 1993; 188:245-248.

89. Parkkola R, Rytokoski U, Kormano M. Magnetic resonance imaging of the discs and trunk muscles in patients with chronic low back pain and healthy control subjects. Spine 1993; 18:830-836.

90. Buirski G, Silberstein M. The symptomatic lumbar disc in patients with low-back pain: Magnetic resonance imaging appearances in both a symptomatic and control population. Spine 1993; 18:1808-1811.

91. Major NM, Helms CA, Genant HK. Calcification demonstrated as high signal intensity on T1-weighted MR images of the disks of the lumbar spine. Radiology 1993; 189:494-496.

92. Ross JS, Ruggieri P, Tkach J, Obuchowski N, Dillinger J, Masaryk TJ, Modic MT. Lumbar degenerative disk disease: Prospective comparison of conventional T2-weighted spin-echo imaging and T2-weighted rapid acquisition relaxation-enhanced imaging. AJNR 1993; 14:1215-1223.

93. Ciricillo SF, Weinstein PR. Lumbar spine stenosis. West J Med 1993; 158:171-177.

94. Schnebel B, Kingston S, Watkins R, et al. Comparison of MRI to CT in the diagnosis of spinal stenosis. Spine 1989; 14:332-337.

95. Gaskill M, Lukin R, Wiot G. Lumbar disc disease and stenosis. Radiol Clin North Am 1991; 29:753-764.

96. Modic MT, Masaryk TJ, Mulopulos GP, et al. Cervical radiculopathy: Prospective evaluation with surface coil MR imaging, CT with metrizamide, and metrizamide myelography. Radiology 1986; 161:753-759.

97. Modic MT, Masaryk TJ, Ross JS, et al. Cervical radiculopathy: value of oblique MR imaging. Radiology 1987; 163:227-331.

98. Hedberg MC, Drayer BP, Flom RA, et al. Gradient echo (GRASS) MR imaging in cervical radiculopathy. AJR 1988; 150:663-689.

99. Van Dyke C, Ors JS, Tkach J, et al. Gradient-echo MR imaging of the cervical spine: Evaluation of extradural disease. Am J Neuroadiol 1989; 10:627-632.

100. Kent DL, Haynor DR, Larson EB, et al. Diagnosis of lumbar spinal stenosis in adults: A metaanalysis of the accuracy of CT, MR, and myelography. Am J Radiol 1992; 158:1135-1144.

101. Rydevik B. Spinal stenosis — conclusions. ACTA Orthop Scand 1993; 64:81-82.

102. Deyo RA. Magnetic resonance imaging of the lumbar spine. [editorial]. N Engl J Med 1994; 331:115-116.

103. Bowen V, Shannon R, Kirkaldy-Willis WH. Lumbar spinal stenosis: A review article. Childs Brain 1978; 4:257-277.

104. Frymoyer JW. Backpain and sciatica. N Engl J Med 1988; 318:291-300.

105. Wiltse LL, Kirkaldy-Willis WH, McIvor GWD. The treatment of spinal stenosis. Clin Orthop 1976; 115:83-91.

106. Kirkaldy-Willis WH, Paine KW, Cauchoix J, et al. Lumbar spinal stenosis. Clin Orthop 1974; 99:30-50.

107. Spengler DM. Degenerative stenosis of the lumbar spine. J Bone Joint Surg (Am) 1987; 69A:305-308.

108. Lee CK, Hansen HT, Weiss AB. Developmental lumbar spinal stenosis: Pathology and surgical treatment. Spine 1978; 3:246-255.

109. Epstein JA, Epstein BJ, Lavine L. Nerve root compression associated with narrowing of the lumbar spinal canal. J Neurol Neurosurg Psychiatry 1962; 25:165-176.

110. Schonstrom NS, Bolender NF, Spengler DM. The pathomorphology of spinal stenosis as seen on CT scans of the lumbar spine. Spine 1985; 10:806-811.

111. Weinstein PR. Diagnosis and management of lumbar spinal stenosis. Clin Neurosurg 1983; 30:677-697.

112. Herkowitz HN, Garlin SR, Bell GR, et al. The use of computerized tomography in evaluating non-visualized vertebral levels caudad to a complete block on a lumbar myelogram, a review of thirty-two cases. J Bone Joint Surg (Am) 1987; 69A:218-224.

113. Quencer RM, Murtagh FR, Post JD, et al. Postoperative bony stenosis of the lumbar spinal canal: Evaluation of 164 symptomatic patients with axial radiography. Am J Roentgenol 1978; 131:1059-1064.

114. Gonzalez EG, Hajdu M, Bruno R, et al. Lumbar spinal stenosis: Analysis of pre- and postoperative somatosensory evoked potentials. Arch Phys Med Rehabil 1985; 66:11-15.

115. McAfee PC, Ullrich CG, Yuan HA, et al. Computed tomography in degenerative spinal stenosis. ACTA Orthop Scand 1981; 52:427-433.

116. Dublin AB, McGahan JP, Reid MH. The value of computed tomographic metrizamide myelography in the neuroradiological evaluation of the spine. Radiology 1983; 146:79-86.

117. Williams DM, Gabrielson TO, Latack JT, et al. Ossification in the cephalic attachment of the ligamentum flavum: An anatomical and CT study. Radiology 1984; 150:423-426.

118. Arroyo IL, Barron KS, Brewer EJ. Spinal cord compression by epidural lipomatosis in juvenile rheumatoid arthritis. Arthritis Rheum 1988; 31:447-451.

119. Urso S, Postacchini F. The value of transverse axial tomography in the diagnosis of lumbar stenosis. Ital J Orthop Traumatol 1978; 4:213-221.

120. Simeone FA, Rothman RH. Clinical usefulness of CT scanning in the diagnosis and treatment of lumbar spine disease. Radiol Clin North Am 1983; 21:197-200.

121. Postacchini F, Petteri G. CT scanning versus myelography in the diagnosis of lumbar stenosis, a preliminary report. Int Orthop 1981; 5:209-215.

122. Lee BCP, Kazam E, Neuman AD. Computed tomography of the spine and spinal cord. Radiology 1978; 128-95–102.

123. Hammerschlag SB, Wolpert SM, Carter BL. Computed tomography of the spinal canal. Radiology 1976; 121:361-367.

124. Burton CV, Kenneth BH, Kirkaldy-Willis W, et al. Computed tomographic scanning and the lumbar spine: II. Clinical considerations. Spine 1978; 4:356-368.

125. Lancourt JE, Glenn WV, Wiltse LL. Multiplanar computerized tomography in the normal spine and in the diagnosis of spinal stenosis. A gross anatomic-computerized tomographic correlation. Spine 1979; 4:379-390.

126. Jacobson RE, Gargano RP, Rosomoff HL. Transverse axial tomography of the spine: 2. The stenotic spinal canal. J Neurosurg 1975; 42:412-419.

127. Keim HA. Diagnostic problems in the lumbar spine. Clin Neurosurg 1979; 25:184-192.

128. Pleatment CW, Lukin RR. Lumbar spinal stenosis. Semin Roentgenol 1988; 23:106-110.

129. Kaiser MC, Capesius P, Roilgen A, et al. Epidural venous stasis in spinal stenosis—CT appearance. Neuroradiology 1985; 26:435-438.

130. Helms CA. CT of the lumbar spine—stenosis and arthrosis. Comput Radiol 1982; 6:359-369.

131. Gaskill MF, Lukin R, Wiot JG. Lumbar disc disease and stenosis. Radiol Clin North Am 1001; 29:753-764.

132. Hyman RA, Merten CW, Liebeskind AL, et al. Computed tomography in ossification of the posterior longitudinal ligament. Neuroradiology 1977; 13:227-228.

133. Crawshaw C, Kean DM, Mulholland RC, et al. The use of nuclear magnetic resonance in the diagnosis of lateral canal entrapment. J Bone Joint Surg (AM) 1984; 66:711-715.

134. Modic MT, Massaryk T, Boumphrey M, et al. Lumbar herniated disk disease and canal stenosis: Prospective evaluation by surface coil MR, CT, and myelography. AJR 1991; 147:757-765.

135. Resnick D. Synovial cysts, Imaging techniques in intraspinal diseases. In Haughton V (ed): Bone and joint imaging. WB Saunders, Philadelphia, 1989, p. 146.

136. Phytinen J, Lahde S, Tanska EL, et al. Computed tomography after lumbar myelography in lower back and extremity pain syndrome. Diagn Imaging 1983; 52:19-22.

137. Ho E, Upadhyay S, Chan F, et al. New methods of measuring vertebral rotation from computed tomographic scans. An intraobserver and interobserver study on girls with scoliosis. Spine 1993; 18(9): 1173-1177.

138. Reinke T, Jahn W. Spinal diagnostic imaging: Computerized axial tomography vs. magnetic resonance imaging. Am J Chiro Med 1988; 1(14):181-184.

139. Brightbill T, Pile N, Eichelberger R, et al. Normal magnetic resonance imaging and abnormal discography in lumbar disc disruption. Spine 1994; 19(9):1075-1077.

140. Brodeur R, Hansmeier D. Variability of intervertebral angle calculations for lateral cervical videofluoroscopic examinations. Proc of the Int'l Conf on Spinal Manip 1993; 37.

141. Byrd R, Kahler J, Leaman S, et al. Reliability of magnetic resonance imaging for morphometry of the intervertebral foramen. Proc of the Int'l Conf on Spinal Manip 1990; 79-82.

142. Cantu J, Cramer G, Dorsett R, et al. Magnetic resonance imaging of the cervical intervertebral foramina: Comparison of two techniques. Proc of the Int'l Conf on Spinal Manip 1994; 101-103.

143. Cramer G, Cantu J, Greenstein J, et al. The accuracy of magnetic resonance imaging in determining the vertical dimensions of the cervical intervertebral foramina. Proc of the Int'l Conf on Spinal Manip 1993; 38-40.

144. Eldevik O, Dugstad G, Orrison W, et al. The effect of clinical bias on the interpretation of myelography and spinal computed tomography. Radiology 1982; 145:85-89.

145. Wallace H, Wagon R, Pierce W. Inter-examiner reliability using videofluoro-scope to measure cervical spine kinematics: A sagittal plane (lateral view). Proc of the Int'l Conf on Spinal Manip 1992; 7-8.

146. Jackson BL, Bunker WF, Bentz J, Gamble AG. Inter and intra examiner relia-bility of upper cervical x-ray marking system: a second look. J Manipulative Physiol Ther, 1987 10:157-63.

147. Seemann DC. A reliability study using positive nasium to establish laterality. The Upper Cervical Monograph, 5(4):7-8.

148. Sigler DC, Howe JW. Inter- and intra examiner reliability of the upper cervi-cal x-ray marking system. J Manipulative Physiol Ther 1985;8:75-80.

149. Grostic JD, DeVoer KP. Roentgenographic measurement of atlas laterality and rotation: a retrospective pre- and post manipulation study. J Manipulative Physiol Ther 1982;5:63-71.

150. Gay RE. The curve of the cervical spine: Variations and significance. J Manipulative Physiol Ther, 199316(9):591-594.

151. Owens EF. Line drawings analyses of static cervical x-ray used in chiroprac-tic. J Manipulative Physiol Ther, 1992; 15:442-449.

152. Rochester RP. Inter and intra-examiner reliability of the upper cervical x-ray marking system: A third and expanded look. Chiropractic Research Journal 1994; 3(1).

153. Plaugher G, Hendricks AH. The interexaminer reliability of the Gonstead pelvic marking system. Proc of the Int'l Conf on Spinal Manip. Arlington, VA, 1990. p. 93-8.

154. Zengel F, Davis BP. Biomechanical analysis by chiropractic radiography: Part II. Effects of x-ray projectional distortion on apparent vertebral rotation. J Manipulative Physiol Ther 1988; 11(5):380-9.

155. Zengel F, Davis BP. Biomechanical analysis by chiropractic radiography: Part III. Lack of effect of projectional distortion on Gonstead vertebral end-plate lines. J Manipulative Physiol Ther 1988; 11(6):469-73.

156. Leach RA. An evaluation of the effect of chiropractic manipulative therapy on hypolordosis of the cervical spine. J Manipulative Physiol Ther 1983; 6(1):17-23.

157. Troyanovich S, Robertson G, Harrison D, Holland B. Intra- and interexaminer reliability of the Chiropractic Biophysics lateral lumbar radiographic mensura-tion procedure. J Manipulative Physiol Ther 1995; 18(8):519-524.

158. Jackson B, Harrison D, Robertson G, Barker W. Chiropractic biophysics lateral cervical film analysis reliability. J Manipulative Physiol Ther 1993; 16(6):384-391.

159. Phillips RV. The use of x-rays in spinal manipulative therapy. In Halderman S (ed) Modern Developments in the Principles and Practice of Chiropractic. Norwalk, CT. Appleton-Century-Crofts, 1980.

160. Buehler MT, Hrejsa AF. Application of lead-acrylic compensating filters in chiropractic full spine radiography: a technical report. J Manipulative Physiol Ther 1985; 8(3):175-80.

161. Shaff AM. Video fluoroscopy as a method of detecting occipitoatlantal instability in Down's syndrome for Special Olympics. Chiropractic Sports Medicine 1994; 8(4):144.

162. Wallace H, Wagnon R, Pierce W. Inter-examiner reliability using videofluoroscope to measure cervical spine kinematics: a sagittal plane (lateral view). Proc of the Int'l Conf on Spinal Manip May 1992:7-8.

163. Van Mameren H, Sanches H, Beursgens J, Drukker J. Cervical spine motion in the sagittal plane II. Spine 1992; 17(5):467.

164. Ochs CW. Radiographic examination of the cervical spine in motion. US Navy Med 1974; 64:21.

165. Buonocard E, Hartman JT, Nelson CL. Cineradiograms of cervical spine in diagnosis of soft-tissue injuries. JAMA 1981(1):143, 1966.

166. Jones MD. Cineradiographic studies of abnormalities of high cervical spine. AMA Arch Surg 1967; 94:206.

167. Tasharski CC. Dynamic atlanto-axial aberration: a case study and cinefluorographic approach to diagnosis. J Manipulative Physiol Ther 1981; 4(2):75.

168. Woesner ME, Mitts MG. The evaluation of cervical spine motion below C-2: a comparison of cineroentgenographic methods. Am J Roent Rad Ther & Nuc Med 1972; 115(1):148.

169. Bard G, Jones MD. Cineradiographic recording of traction of the cervical spine. Arch Phys Med 1964; 45:403.

170. Bard G, Jones MD. Cineradiographic analysis of laminectomy in cervical spine. AMA Arch Surg 1968; 97;672.

171. Brunton FJ, Wilkerson JA, Wise KS, Simonis RB. Cineradiography in cervical spondylosis as a means of determining the level for anterior fusion. J Bone Joint Surg 1982; 64-B(4):399.

172. Jones MD. Cineradiographic studies of collar immobilized cervical spine. J Neurosurg 1960; 17;633.

173. Jones MD. Cineradiographic studies of various joint diseases in the cervical spine. Arthritis & Rheumatism 1961; 4:422.

174. Jones MD. Cineradiographic studies of degenerative disease of the cervical spine. J Canad Assoc Radiol 1961; 12:52.

175. Jones MD, Stone BS, Bard G. Occipitalization of atlas with hypoplastic odontoid process, a cineroentgenographic study. Calif Med 1966; 104:309.

176. Gillet H. A cineradiographic study of the kinetic relationship between the cervical vertebrae. Bull Eur Chiro Union 1980; 28(3):44.

177. Henderson DJ. Kinetic roentgenographic analysis of the cervical spine in the saggital plane: a preliminary study. Int Review of Chiro 1981; 35:2.

178. Howe JW. Observations from cineroentgenological studies of the spinal column. ACA J of Chiro 1970; 7(10: 75.

179. Leung ST. The value of cineradiographic motion studies in diagnosis of dysfunctions of the cervical spine. Bull Eur Chiro Union 1977; 25(2):28.

180. Shippel AH, Robinson GK. Radiological and magnetic resonance imaging of the cervical spine instability: A case report. J Manipulative Physiol Ther 1987; 10(6):316.

181. Antos J. Robinson GK, Keating JC, Jacobs GE. Interexaminer reliability of cinefluoroscopic detection of fixation in the mid-cervical spine. Proceedings of the Scientific Symposium on Spinal Biomechanics, International Chiropractors Association, 1989, p. 41.

182. Taylor M, Skippings R. Paradoxical motion of atlas in flexion: a fluoroscopic study of chiropractic patients. Euro J Chiro 1987; 35:116.

183. Betge G. The value of cineradiographic motion studies in the diagnosis of dysfunction of the cervical spine. J Clin Chiro 1979; 2(6):40.

184. Masters B. A cineradiographic study of the kinetic relationship between the cervical vertebrae. Bull Eur Chiro Union 1980; 28(1):11.

185. Mertz JA. Videofluoroscopy of the cervical and lumbar spine. ACA J Chiro 1981; 18(8):74.

186. Robinson GK. Interpretation of videofluoroscopic joint motion studies in the cervical spine C-2 to C-7. The Verdict, February 1988.

187. Akeson WH, Woo SL, Taylor TK, Ghosh P, Bushell GR. Biomechanics and biochemistry of the intervertebral discs. Clin Orthop 1977; (122):133.

188. White AA, Johnson RM, Panjabi MM, Southwick WO. Biomechanical analysis of clinical stability in the cervical spine. Clin Orthop 1975; (109):85.

189. Vernon H. Static and dynamic roentgenography in the diagnosis of degenerative disc disease: a review and comparative assessment. J Manipulative Physiol Ther 1982; 5(4):163.

190. Ressel OJ. Disc regeneration: reversibility is possible in spinal osteoarthritis. ICA Review 1989; 45(2):39.

191. Posner I, White AA, Edwards WT, Hayes WC. A biomechanical analysis of the clinical stability of the lumbar and lumbosacral spine. Spine 1982; 7:374.

192. Nachemson A. Towards a better understanding of low back pain; a review of the mechanics of the lumbar disc. Rheumatol Rehabil 1975; 14(3):129.

193. Huelke DF, Nusholtz GS. Cervical spine biomechanics: a review of the literature. J Orthop Res 1986; 4(2):232.

194. Karnaze MG, Gado MH, Sartos KJ, Hodges FJ 3d. Comparison of MR and CT myelography in imaging the cervical and thoracic spine. AJR 1988; 150(2):397.

195. Kulkarni MV, Narayana PA, McArdle CB, Yeakley JW, et al. Cervical spine MR imaging using multislice gradient echo imaging: comparison with cardiac gated spin echo. Magn Reson Imaging 1988; 6(5):517.

196. Takahashi M, Sakamoto Y, Miyawaki M, Bussaka H. Increased MR signal intensity secondary to chronic cervical cord compression. Neuroradiology 1987; 29(6):550.

197. Grenier N, Kressel HY, Scheibler ML, Grossman RI, Dalinka M. Normal and degenerative posterior spinal structures: MR Imaging. Radiology 1987; 165(2):517.

198. Richards G, Thompson J, Osterbauer T, Fuhr A. Use of pre- and post-CT scans and clinical findings to monitor low force chiropractic care of patients with sciatic neuropathy and lumbar disc herniation: A review. J Manipulative Physiol Ther 1990, 13:58.

199. Walker B. The use of computer-assisted tomography of the lumbar spine in a chiropractic practice. Journal of the Australian Chiropractic Association 1985; 15:86.

200. Koentges A. Computerized axial tomography of the spine in the differential diagnosis of vertebral subluxations. Annals of the Swiss Chiropractors' Association 1985; 8:25.

201. Kent C. Contemporary technologies for imaging the vertebral subluxation complex. ICA Review 1989; 45(4):45.

202. Aldrete JA. Diagnostic ultrasound in pain management: an overview. Am J Pain Management 1994; 4(4):160.

203. Anderson DJ, Adcock DF, Chovil AC, Farrell JJ. Ultrasound lumbar canal measurement in hospital employees with back pain. Br J Ind Med 1988; 45(8):552.

204. Chovil AC, Anderson DJ, Adcock DF. Ultrasonic measurement of lumbar canal diameter: a screening tool for low back disorders? South Med J 1989; 82(8):977.

205. Engel JM, Engel GM, Gunn DR. Ultrasound of the spine in focal stenosis and disc disease. Spine 1985; 10(10):928.

206. Suzuki S, Yamamuro T, Shikata J, Shimizu K, Iida H. Ultrasound measurement of vertebral rotation in idiopathic scoliosis. J Bone Joint Surg 1989; 72-B(2):252.

207. Moore RE. Blind study: comparison of sonographic results in patients with back pain previously diagnosed by MRI, x-ray and standard orthopedic exam. American Journal of Clinical Chiropractic May 1995; 5(2):34.

208. Mandell G. Radionuclide imaging. In: Kricun ME. Imaging modalities in spinal disorders. W.B. Saunders Company, Philadelphia, PA. 1988.

209. Bates D, Ruggieri P. Imaging modalities for evaluation of the spine. Radiologic Clinics of North America 1991;29(4):675-690.

210. Carmichael, J. Clinical case reports in the use of computed tomography for the quantification of leg length inequality. The CT Scanogram. Proc of the Int'l Conf on Spinal Manip. FCER, Arlington, VA. 191, April 1991.

211. Cramer G, Howe J, Glenn W, et al. Comparison of computed tomography to magnetic resonance imaging in evaluation of the intervertebral foramen. Proc of the Int'l Conf on Spinal Manip. FCER, Arlington, VA. 186, 1991.

212. Dreyer P, Lantz CA. Chiropractic management of herniated disc restoration of disc protrusion and management of disc integrity as substantiated by MRI. Proc of the Int'l Conf on Spinal Manip. FCER, Arlington VA. 57, 1991.

213. Richards G, Thompson J, Osterbauer P, et al. Use of pre-and post CT scans and clinical findings to monitor low force chiropractic care of patients with sciatic neuropathy and lumbar disc herniation: A Review. J Manipulative Physiol Ther 1990; 13(1):58.

214. Antos J, Robinson K, Keating J, et al. Interrater reliability of fluoroscopic detection of fixation in the mid-cervical spine. Chiropractic Technique 1990; 2(2):53-55.

215. Krishnamurthy GT, Blahd WH. Technetium-99m polyphosphate bone image for early detection of skeletal metastasis. Correlation with other diagnostic parameters. Nucl Med (Stuttg) 1975; 13(4):330-40.

216. Wetzel LH, Engelbrecht DE, Baxter KG, et al. Comparison of MR imaging and bone scintigraphy for detection and evaluation of osseous spinal metastases. Nineteenth Annual Meeting of the American Roentgen Ray Society. May 13-18, 1990, Washington, DC.

217. Hardy JG, Newble GM. The detection of bone lesions using 99Tcm labelled polyphosphate. Bronchitis J Radiol 1974; 47(563):769-74.

218. Patton DD, Woolfenden JM. Radionuclide bone scanning in diseases of the spine. Radiol Clin North Am 1977; 15(2):177-201.

219. Yamaguchi The, Tamai K, Yamoto M, et al. Intertrabecular pattern of tumors metastatic to bone. Cancer 1996; 78(7):1388-94.

220. Gillet H. A cineradiographic study of the kinematic relationship between the cervical vertebrae. Bull Euro Chiro Union 1980; 28(3):44-46.

221. Pasto ME, Goldberg BB. Chapter 15—Sonography. In Kricun ME: Imaging modalities in spinal disorders. W.B. Saunders Co. New York, NY. 1988.

222. Porter RW, Hilbert C, Wellman P. Backache and the lumbar spinal canal. Spine 1980; 5(2):99.

4 Clinical Impression and Assessment

RECOMMENDATION

Practitioners should develop a method of patient assessment which includes a sufficient diversity of findings to support the clinical impression as related to vertebral subluxation.[1-24] In this regard, it is considered inappropriate to render an opinion regarding the appropriateness of chiropractic care without a chiropractic assessment, including a physical examination of the patient by a licensed chiropractor. When management of patient care is carried out in the collaborative setting, the chiropractor, as a primary contact health care provider, is the only professional qualified to determine the appropriateness of chiropractic care. The unique role of the chiropractor is separate from other health disciplines,[25-35] and should be clarified for both the patient and other practitioners. The patient assessment, specific to the technique practiced by the chiropractor, should minimally include a biomechanical and neurophysiological component. It is inappropriate to make a retrospective determination of the clinical need for care rendered prior to the assessment.

Rating: Established
Evidence: E, L

Commentary

The procedures employed in the chiropractic assessment may include some or all of, but are not limited to the following:

Physical examination:
Palpation (static osseous, static muscle, motion).
Range of motion.
Postural examination
Comparative leg length (static, flexed, cervical syndrome).
Manual muscle tests.
Nerve function tests.
Mental status examination and psychosocial assessment.

Instrumentation examination:
Range of motion.
Thermography.
Temperature reading instruments.
Muscle testing.
Electromyography.
Pressure algometry.
Nerve-function tests.
Electroencephalography and brain mapping.

Bilateral and four quadrant weight scales.

Imaging examination:
Spinography.
Videofluoroscopy.
Computerized tomography.
Magnetic resonance imaging.

Following the determination of a clinical impression, the patient should be made aware of the findings and consent to the proposed plan of care.

Literature support for the use of these technologies may be found in the chapters on chiropractic examination, instrumentation and diagnostic imaging (Chapters 1, 2, 3).

References

1. Leboeuf C, Gardner V, Carter A, et al. Chiropractic examination procedures: A reliability and consistency study. J Aust Chiro Assoc 1989; 19(3):101-104.

2. Mior S, McGregor M, Schut B. The role of experience in clinical accuracy. J Manipulative Physiol Ther 1990; 13(2):68-71.

3. Rhudy T, Sandefur M, Burk J. Interexaminer/intertechnique reliability in spinal subluxation assessment: A multifactorial approach. Am J Chiro Med 1988; 1(3):111-114.

4. Sandefur, R. .Interexaminer/intertechnique reliability in spinal subluxation assessment: A multifactorial approach. Am J Chiro Med 1989; 2(3):131.

5. Upledger, J. The reproducibility of craniosacral examination findings: A statistical analysis. J Am Osteopath Assoc 1977; 76(12):889-890.

6. Damron, D. A retrospective consecutive case analysis of pretreatment and comparative static radiological parameters following chiropractic adjustments. J Manipulative Physiol Ther 1991; 14(5): 334-335.

7. Plaugher G, Cremata E, Phillips R. A retrospective consecutive case analysis of pretreatment and comparative static radiological parameters following chiropractic adjustments. J Manipulative Physiol Ther 1990; 13(9): 498-506.

8. Terrett A. It is more important to know when not to adjust. Chiro Tech 1990; 2(1): 1-9.

9. Adair I, Vanwijk M, Armstrong G. Moiré topography in scoliosis screening. Clin Orthop 1977; (129): 165-171.

10. Ardran G, Dickson R, Dixon-Brown B, et al. Assessment of scoliosis in children: low dose radiographic technique. BR J Radiol 1980; 53:146-147.

11. Osterbauer P, Fuhr A, Hildebrandt R. Mechanical force, manually assisted short lever chiropractic adjustment. J Manipulative Physiol Ther 1992; 15:309-317.

12. Rosen, M. Short lever specific contact procedures. Transactions of the Consortium for Chiropractic Research 1991; 261-264.

13. Burke EJ, Glick D, Grostic J, et al. Validity of selected measures of the DDSSEP protocol: A factor analytic approach. J Manipulative Physiol Ther 1994; 17(4):273.

14. Fisher, AA. Pressure threshold meter: Its use for quantification of tender spots. Arch Phys Med Rehab 1986; 67(11):836-838.

15. Fisher, AA. Tissue compliance meter for objective documentation of soft tissue consistency and pathology. Arch Phys Med Rehab 1987; 68:122-125.

16. Hospers LA, Sweat RW; Hus L, et al. Response of a three year old epileptic child to upper cervical adjustment. Today's Chiro 1987; 15(16):69-76.

17. Jansen R, Nansel D, Slosberg M. Normal paraspinal tissue compliance: The reliability of a new clinical and experimental instrument. J Manipulative Physiol Ther 1990; 13(5):243-246.

18. Wagnon, R. Finally, an objective instrument for assessing the effects of chiropractic intervention. Am Chiro 1991; 13(2):20-22.

19. La Francis, M. A chiropractic perspective of atlantoaxial instability in Down's syndrome. J Manipulative Physiol Ther 1990; 13(3):157-160.

20. Whittingham W, Ellis W, Molyneux T. The effects of manipulation (toggle recoil technique) for headaches with upper cervical joint dysfunction: A pilot study. J Chiro 1994; 17(6):369-375.

21. Hsieh C, Pringle R. Range of motion of the lumbar spine required for four activities of daily living. J Manipulative Physiol Ther 1994; 17(6):353-358.

22. Lea R, Gerhardt J. Range-of-motion measurements. J Bone Joint Surgery 1995; 77A(5):784-798.

23. Nilsson N. Measuring passive cervical motion: A study of reliability. J Manipulative Physiol Ther 1995; 18(5):293-297.

24. Williamson S. Effect of unilateral spinal adjustments on goniometrically-assessed cervical lateral-flexion end-range asymmetries in otherwise asymptomatic subjects. J Manipulative Physiol Ther 1990; 13(7):418.

25. Leach RA. The chiropractic theories: A synopsis of chiropractic research, 2nd ed. Williams & Wilkins, Baltimore, MD, 1986.

26. Palmer DD. The science, art and philosophy of chiropractic. Published by the author, Portland, OR, 1910.

27. Palmer BJ. The science of chiropractic. Palmer School of Chiropractic, Davenport, IA, 1920.

28. Jamison J. Chiropractic as conventional health care. J Aust Chiro Assoc 1989; 15(2):55-59.

29. Janse J. Chiropractic and children. J Can Chiro Assoc 1979; 23(3).

30. Ressel OJ. Chiropractic and children: A rationale for care. Intl Rev Chiro 1986; 42:44-50.

31. Schneier M, Burns R. Atlanto-occipital hypermobility in sudden infant death syndrome. Chiropractic (J Chiro Res Clin Inves) 1991; 7(2):33-38.

32. Vear H. The role of chiropractic in preventive health care. J Can Chiro Assoc 1974; 18(4):10-3.

33. Webster LL. Subluxation at birth and early childhood. Int'l Chiro Pediatric Assoc, Stone Mountain, GA, 1989.

34. Sawyer C, Bergmann T, Good D. Attitudes and habits of chiropractors concerning referral to other health care providers. J Manipulative Physiol Ther 1988; 11:480-483.

35. Seventh Report to the President & Congress on the Status of Health Personnel. U.S. Dept. of Health and Human Services, 1990.

5 Reassessment and Outcomes Assessment

RECOMMENDATION

Determination of the patient's progress must be made on a per-visit and periodic basis. This process provides quantitative and qualitative information regarding the patient's progress which is utilized to determine the frequency and duration of chiropractic care. Per-visit reassessment should include at least one analytical procedure previously used. This chosen testing procedure should be performed each time the patient receives chiropractic care.

Concomitant with this process, the effectiveness of patient care may also be monitored through the development of an outcomes assessment plan. Such a plan may utilize data from the patient examination, assessment and reassessment procedures. Patient-reported quality of life instruments, mental health surveys, and general health surveys are encouraged as part of the outcomes assessment plan. The analysis of data from these sources may be used to change or support continuation of a particular regimen of patient care and/or change or continue the operational procedures of the practice.

Rating: Established
Evidence: E, L

Commentary

The reassessment provides information to determine the necessity of an adjustment on a per-visit basis. Partial reassessment involves duplication of two or more preceding positive analytical procedures. Full reassessment involves duplication of three or more preceding positive analytical procedures. Any additional or complementary analytical procedures should be performed as indicated by the patient's clinical status. The frequency of partial and full reassessments should be at the discretion of the practitioner, consistent with the objectives of the plan of care.

A substantial body of literature attests to the methods and significance of measuring outcomes.[1-100] For the practicing chiropractor the implication is that regular evaluations of practice and procedures provides a form of quality control. Outcomes assessments can alert the practitioner to problems with, as well as reinforce, aspects of practice which might otherwise be overlooked. In addition, ongoing evaluation provides information about the clinical value of care to both patients and third-party providers. It is important to point out that there is no one "ideal" way to assess outcomes. While the responsibility to conduct this type of assessment rests with the chiropractor, so does the choice of how it is to be implemented.

References

1. Mrozek J, Wiles M. A reliability assessment of four-quadrant weight-scale measurements. J Can Chiro Assoc 1982; 26(3):97-100.

2. Deboer K, Harmon R, Savole S, Tuttle C. Inter- and intra-examiner reliability of leg-length differential measurement: A preliminary study. J Manip Physiol Ther 1983; 6(2):61-66.

3. Sandoz R. The choice of appropriate clinical criteria for assessing the progress of a chiropractic case. Annals Swiss Chiro Assoc 1985; 8:53-73.

4. Homewood A. A posturometer survey. J Can Chiro Assoc 1964; 9(1):9-10.

5. Beech R. The fundamentals of the short-leg syndrome. Annals Swiss Chiro Assoc 1965; 3:7-36.

6. Mears D. Spinal analysis. Digest Chiro Econ 1973; 16(3):80-81.

7. Mears D. Analysis of lateral cervical x-ray. Digest Chiro Econ 1972; 14(4):36-37.

8. Pierce W, Stillwagon G. Charting and interpreting skin temperature differential patterns. Digest Chiro Econ 1970; 12(5):37-39.

9. Gillet H. A cineradiographic study of the kinematic relationship between the cervical vertebrae. Bull Euro Chiro Union 1980; 28(3):44-46.

10. Johnston L. Three dimensional spinal analysis: The key to statistical research and public service. Digest Chiro Econ 1967; 10(2):18-19.

11. Brunarski D. Chiropractic biomechanical evaluations: Validity in myofascial low back pain. J Manipulative Physiol Ther 1982; 5(4):155-160.

12. Dailey E, Buehler M. Plain film assessment of spinal stenosis: method comparison with lumbar CT. J Manipulative Physiol Ther 1989; 12:192-199.

13. Kobrossi T, Schut B. The use of the objective structured clinic examination (OSCE) at the Canadian Memorial Chiropractic College Outpatient Clinic. J Can Chiro Assoc 1987; 31:21-25.

14. Richards D, Thompson J, Osterbauer P, Fuhr A. Use of pre- and post-CT scans and clinical findings to monitor low force chiropractic care of patients with sciatic neuropathy and lumbar disc herniations: A review. J Manipulative Physiol Ther 1990; 13(1):58.

15. Hsieh C, Phillips R. Reliability of manual muscle testing, with a computerized dynamometer. J Manipulative Physiol Ther 1990; 13(2):72-82.

16. McGregor M, Minor S. Anatomical and functional perspectives of the cervical spine: Part I: The "normal" cervical spine. J Can Chiro Assoc 1989; 33:123-129.

17. Jansen R, Nansel D, Slosberg M. Normal paraspinal tissue compliance: the reliability of a new clinical and experimental instrument. J Manipulative Physiol Ther 1990; 13(5):243-246.

18. Herbert S. Computer graphics research in chiropractic comes of age. ICA Rev Chiro 1985; 25-27.

19. Hildebrandt R. Chiropractic spinography and postural roentgenology — Part I: History of development. J Manipulative Physiol Ther 1980; 3(2):87-92.

20. Christensen K. Medical vs. chiropractic x-ray interpretation. Am Chiro 1982; 20-23.

21. Kent C, Gentempo P, Grostic J, Grassam I, Gregg R, Hofmann J. A consensus approach to subluxation-based chiropractic: Phase I questionnaire results.

22. Kent C, Gentempo P. The documentary basis for diagnostic imaging procedures in the subluxation-based chiropractic practice. ICA, Arlington, VA, 1992.

23. Wallace H, Pierce WV, Wagnon R. Cervical flexion and extension analysis using digitized videofluoroscopy. Chiropractic: J Chiro Research and Clinical Investigation 1992; 7(4):94-97.

24. Adams A, Loper D, Willd S, Lawless P, Loueks J. Intra- and interexaminer reliability of plumb line posture analysis measurements using a 3-dimensional electrogoniometer. Res For 1988; 4(3):60-72.

25. Boline PD, Keating JC, Brist J, Denver G. Interexaminer reliability of palpatory evaluations of the lumbar spine. Am J Chiro Med 1988; 1(1):5-11.

26. Beal M, Vorro J, Johnson W. Chronic cervical dysfunction: correlation of myoelectric findings with clinical progress. J Am Osteopath Assoc 1989; 89:391-900.

27. Becker R. The body electric: electromagnetism and the foundation of life. Quill, NY, 1985.

28. BenEliyahu DJ. Thermographic imaging of pathoneurophysiology due to cervical disc herniation. J Manipulative Physiol Ther 1989; 12:482-490.

29. Brieg A, Turnbull I, Hassler C. Effect of mechanical stresses on the spinal cord in cervical spondylosis. J Neurosurg 1966; 25:45-56.

30. Brighton P, Graham R, Bird H. Hypermobility of the joints. Springer-Verlag, NY, 1983.

31. Carmichael J. Clinical case reports in the use of computed tomography for the quantification of leg length inequality: The CT scanogram. Proc of the Int'l Conf on Spinal Manip. FCER, Arlington, VA 1991; 191.

32. Chang-Yu J, Hsieh DC, Phillips EB, Adams A, Pope MH. Functional outcomes of low back pain: comparison of four treatment groups in a randomized controlled trial. J Manipulative Physiol Ther 1992; 15(1):4-10.

33. Cherkin DC. Patient satisfaction as an outcome measure. J Chiropractic Tech 1990; 2(3):138.

34. Cooperstein R, Gardner R, Hansel D. Concordance of two methods of motion palpation with goniometrically-assessed cervical lateral flexion asymmetry. Proc of the Int'l Conf on Spinal Manip. FCER, Arlington, VA 1991; 186.

35. Cram J. Clinical EMG: muscle scanning for surface recordings. Biofeedback Inst of Seattle, Seattle, WA, 1986.

36. Cramer G, Howe J, Glenn W, Greenstein J, Marx P, Johnson S, Huntoon R, Cantu J, Emde J, Aoys M. Comparison of computed tomography to magnetic resonance imaging in evaluation of the intervertebral foramen. Proc of the Int'l Conf on Spinal Manip. FCER, Arlington, VA 1991; 186.

37. Deyo RA. Measuring the functional status of patients with low back pain. J Chiropractic Tech 1990; 2(3):127.

38. Diakow P. Thermographic assessment of sacroiliac syndrome: report of a case. J Can Chiro Assoc 1990; 34(3):131.

39. Dreyer P, Lantz CA. Chiropractic management of herniated disc. Restoration of disc protrusion and management of disc integrity as substantiated by MRI. Proc of the Int'l Conf on Spinal Manip. FCER, Arlington, VA 1991; 57.

40. Eddy J. Designing a practice policy: standards, guidelines, options and clinical decision making. JAMA 1990; 263(2):3077.

41. Ellwood P. Outcomes management: a technology of patient experience. N Engl J Med 1988; 318:23.

42. Flesia J. The vertebral subluxation complex: an integrative perspective. ICA Intl Rev Chiro 1992; 25.

43. Granger M, McDowell S. An investigation of the effect of chiropractic treatment upon the mobility of the spine. Eur J Chiro 1985; 33(3):143-164.

44. Grostic J. Roentgenographic measurement of Atlas laterality and rotation: a retrospective pre- and post-manipulation study. J Manipulative Physiol Ther 1982; 5(2):63.

45. Haas M, Nylendo J. Lumbar motion trends and correlation with low back pain. A roentgenographic evaluation and quantitative segmental motion in lateral bending. Proc 1991 World Chiro Congr Toronto, 1991.

46. Haas M, Nylendo J. Diagnostic utility of the McGill questionnaire and the Oswestry Disability questionnaire for classification of low back pain syndrome. J Manipulative Physiol Ther 1992; 15(22):90-98.

47. Haldeman S. Spinal manipulation therapy in the management of low back pain. HE Finnegan (ed), Lippincott, Toronto, 1973.

48. Hansen D. Development and use of clinical algorithms in chiropractic. J Manip Physiol Ther 1991; 14(8):478-482.

49. Gerzog W, Conway P, Willcox B. Effects of different treatment modalities on gait symmetry and clinical measures for sacroiliac joint patients. J Manipulative Physiol Ther 1991; 14(2):104-109.

50. Homewood AE. The neurodynamics of the vertebral subluxation complex, 3rd ed. Valkyrie Press, St. Petersburg, FL, 1977.

51. Hsieh J, Phillips R. Reliability of manual muscle testing with a computerized dynamometer. J Manipulative Physiol Ther 1990; 13(2):72.

52. Hsieh CY. Instrumentation of reported low back pain clinical trials. Proc 1989 Intl Conf on Spinal Manip 2-14, 1989.

53. Jaeschke R, Singer J, Guyatt G. A comparison of seven-point and visual analog scales: data from a randomized trial. Controlled Clin Trials 1990; 11:43-51.

54. Jansen R, Nansel D, Slosbert M. Normal paraspinal compliance. The reliability of a new clinical experimental instrument. J Manipulative Physiol Ther 1990; 13(5):243.

55. Jirout J. Studies of the dynamics of the spine. Acta Rad 1956; 4655-60.

56. Jose W. Outcome measures for chiropractic health care, Part I: introduction to outcomes assessment and general health assessment instruments. Spinal Manip 1991; 7(22):1-5.

57. Kapandji IA. The physiology of joints, Vol III. LH Honore (trans). Churchill Livingstone, New York, NY, 1974.

58. Keating JC. Rationalism and empiricism vs. the philosophy of science in chiropractic. Chiro Hist 1990; 10(2):23.

59. Kent C, Gentempo P. The documentary basis for diagnostic imaging procedures in the subluxation-based chiropractic practice. ICA 1992.

60. Kirkaldy-Willis W, Yong-Hong K, Reilly J. Pathology and pathogenesis of lumbar spondylosis and stenosis. Spine 1978; 3(4):319.

61. Koss I. The spinal cord as organizer of disease, Process I. J Am Osteo Assoc 1976; 76(1):34-35.

62. Korr I. The peripheral nervous system, II. J Am Osteo Assoc 1979; 79(2):82-90.

63. Lawlis G, Cuencas R, Selby D, McCoy C. The development of the Dallas Pain questionnaire: an assessment of the impact of spinal pain on behavior. Spine 1989; 14(5):511-516.

64. Lovell F, Rothstein J, Personius W. Reliability of clinical measurements of lumbar lordosis taken with a flexible rule. Phys Ther 1989; 69(2):96-105.

65. Manello D. Leg length inequality: a review. Proc Sixth Annual Conf on Research and Education. Consortium for Chiro Res, 1990.

66. McLachlan C. Enhanced patient decision-making: a role for outcomes management systems. Proc Intl Conf on Spinal Manip. FCER, Arlington, VA 1991; 3.

67. Meade TW, Dyer S, Browne W, Townsend J, Frank AO. Low back pain of mechanical origin: randomized comparison of chiropractic and hospital outpatient treatment. Brit Med J 1990; 300(6737):1437.

68. Meeker W, Gahlinger P. Neuromuscular thermography: a valuable diagnostic tool? J Manipulative Physiol Ther 1986; 9:257-266.

69. Miol S, Grockman J, Fournier G, Vernon H. A comparison of two objective measures in assessing cervical range of motion. Proc of the Int'l Conf on Spinal Manip. FCER, Arlington, VA 1991; 79-81.

70. Nansel DD, Peneff A, Quitoriano J. Effectiveness of upper vs. lower cervical adjustments with respect to the amelioration of passive rotational vs. lateral-flexion end-range asymmetries in otherwise asymptomatic subjects. J Manipulative Physiol Ther 1992; 15(2):99-105.

71. Nylendo J, Haas M, Jones R. Using the SF-36D (General Health Questionnaire) in a pilot study of outcome assessment for low back chiropractic patients. Proc of the Int'l Conf on Spinal Manip. FCER, Arlington, VA 1991; 172.

72. Panjabi MM, White A, Brand R. A note on defining body part configurations. J Biomech 1974; 7:385.

73. Plaugher G. Skin temperature assessment for neuromuscular abnormalities of the spinal column: a review. Proc 6th Annual Conf on Research and Education, June 21-23, 1991.

74. Robinson R, Herzog W, Nigg B. Use of force platform variables to quantify the effects of chiropractic manipulation on gait symmetry. J Manipulative Physiol Ther 1987; 19(4):172-176.

75. Russell G, Raso V, Hill D, McIvor J. A comparison of four computerized methods for measuring vertebral rotation. Spine 1990; 15(1):24-27.

76. Sandoz R. Some physical mechanisms and effects of spinal adjustments . Ann Swiss Chiro Assoc 1976; 6(2):91-142.

77. Sawyer C. Patient satisfaction as a chiropractic research outcome. Proc of the Int'l Conf on Spinal Manip. FCER, Arlington, VA 1991;163, Apr,.

78. Schafer R, Faye L. Motion palpation and chiropractic technique. Principles of dynamic chiropractic. Motion Palp Instrument, Huntington Beach, CA, 1981.

79. Sharpless SK. Susceptibility of spinal roots to compression block. Res Status of Spinal Manip Ther. Washington, NIH Workshop, NINCDS Monograph 1975; 15:155-161.

80. Suh CH. Researching the fundamentals of chiropractic. J Bio Conf Spine. U of Colo. 1974; 5:1-52.

81. Thabe J. Electromyography as tool to document diagnostic findings and therapeutic results associated with somatic dysfunction in the upper cervical spinal joints and sacro-iliac joints. Manual Med 1986; 2:53-58.

82. Wallace H, Clapper J., Wood J, Wagnon R. A method for measuring changes in cervical flexion and extension using videofluoroscopy. Proc of the Int'l Conf on Spinal Manip. FCER, Arlington, VA 1991; 175-182.

83. Vernon H. Applying research based assessments of pain and loss of function to the issue of developing standards of care in chiropractic. J Chiropractic Tech 1990; 2(3):121.

84. Diener E, Suh E, Smith H, et al. National differences in reported subjective well-being: why do they occur? Social Indicators Research 1995; 34:7-32.

85. Grant M, Ferrell B, Schmidt GM, et al. Measurement of quality of life in bone marrow transplantation survivors. Quality of Life Research 1992; 1:375-384.

86. Barrett S. Complementary self-care strategies for healthy aging. Generations 1993; 17(3)49.

87. Clouser KD, Hufford D. Nonorthodox healing systems and their knowledge claims. The Journal of Medicine and Philosophy 1993; 18(2)101-106.

88. Wilson I, Cleary P. Linking clinical variables with health-related quality of life. A conceptual model of patient outcome. JAMA 1995; 273(1)59-65.

89. Kenney J. The consumer's views of health. Journal of Advanced Nursing 1992; 17(7)829-834.

90. Pavot W, Diener E. The affective and cognitive context of self-reported measures of subjective well-being. Social Indicators Research 1993; 28:1-20.

91. Diener E. Assessing subjective well-being: progress and opportunities. Social Indicators Research 1994; 31:103-157.

92. Boone WR, Dobson GJ. A proposed vertebral subluxation model reflecting traditional concepts and recent advances in health and science: Part III. Journal Vertebral Subluxation Research 1997; 1(3):25-33.

93. Franklin G, Haug J, Heyer N. Outcome of lumbar fusion in Washington State Worker's Compensation. Spine 1994; 19(17)1897-1904.

94. Glick D, Lee F, Grostic J. Documenting the efficacy of chiropractic care utilizing somatosensory evoked potential (SEP) testing: Post spinal adjustment changes in SEPs. Proc of the Int'l Conf on Spinal Manip A/M 1993; 82.

95. Hagino C, Papernick L. Test-retest reliability of the 'CMCC low back status questionnaire for laypersons'. Proc of the Intl Conf on Spinal Manip A/M 1993; 47.

96. Hains F, Waalen J, Mior S. Psychometric properties of the Neck Disability Index; final results. Proc of the Int'l Conf on Spinal Manip 1994; 8-9.

97. Hawk C, Wallace H, Dusio M. Development of a global well-being scale: A study of reliability, validity and responsiveness. Proc of the Int'l Conf on Spinal Manip 1994; 41-42.

98. Liang M, Andersson G, Bombardier C, et al. Strategies for outcome research in spinal disorders. Spine 1994; 19(18S)2037S-2040S.

99. Whitton M. Outcomes assessment: its relationship to chiropractic and managed health care. J Chiro 1994; 31(7)37-40.

100. Stano M. A comparison of health care costs for chiropractic and medical patients. J Manipulative Physiol Ther 1993. 16:291-299.

6 Modes of Adjustive Care

RECOMMENDATION

Adjusting procedures should be selected which are determined by the practitioner to be safe and effective for the individual patient. No mode of care should be used which has been demonstrated by critical scientific study and field experience to be unsafe or ineffective in the correction of vertebral subluxation.

Rating: Established

Evidence: E, L

Commentary

This chapter is concerned with the modes of adjustive care (techniques) associated with the correction of vertebral subluxation. The literature reveals many articles on adjusting modes. These articles include technique descriptions, various applications of techniques, and reliability studies usually assessing inter- and intra-examiner reliability. A number of review articles provide discussion of the modes of care. Available research data has been complemented with professional opinion, derived from two separate forums of chiropractic experts' The International Straight Chiropractic Consensus Conference, Chandler, Arizona (1992) and the Council on Chiropractic Practice Symposium on Chiropractic Techniques, Phoenix, Arizona, (1996), both of which served to validate procedures by common knowledge and usage.

The intent of this chapter is not to include nor exclude any particular technique, but rather to provide a guideline, drawing upon the commonality of various techniques, which contributes to the chiropractic objective of correcting vertebral subluxation. Any technique which does not espouse the correction of subluxation would be considered outside the scope of the Guidelines.

A list of descriptive terms and definitions related to chiropractic adjustive care as commonly practiced follows:

Adjustment: The correction of a vertebral subluxation.

Adjustic Thrust: The specific application of force to facilitate the correction of vertebral subluxation.

Adjusting Instruments: Fixed or hand-held mechanical instruments used to deliver a specific, controlled thrust to correct a vertebral subluxation.

Amplitude: Magnitude; greatness of size or depth.

Blocking Technique: The use of mechanical leverage, achieved through positioning of the spine or related structures, to facilitate the correction of vertebral subluxation.

Cleavage: The movement of one vertebra between two other vertebrae.

Concussion: An adjustic thrust produced by arrested momentum. Momentum is the result of weight (mass) in motion and also of speed. An adjustic concussion depends more on speed than mass.

High Velocity Thrust with Recoil: A controlled thrust delivered such that the time of impact with the vertebra coincides with the chiropractor's contact recoil, thus setting the vertebra in a specific directional motion.

Impulse: A sudden force directionally applied to correct a malpositioned joint.

Low Velocity Thrust with Recoil: A controlled thrust administered at low speed with a sudden pull-off by the practitioner, setting the segment in motion.

Low Velocity Thrust without Recoil: A controlled thrust administered at low speed coupled with a sustained contact on the segment adjusted.

Low Velocity Vectored Force without Recoil: A short or long duration (usually ranging from 1 to 20 seconds) contact with the segment being adjusted, with or without a graduation of force.

Manually Assisted Mechanical Thrust: A manually delivered specific thrust enhanced by a moving mechanism built into the adjusting table.

Manipulation: The taking of a joint past its passive range of motion into the paraphysiological space but not past the anatomic limit, accompanied by articular cavitation (Kirkaldy-Willis). It is not synonymous with chiropractic adjustment, which is applied to correct vertebral subluxation.

Multiple Impulse: Impulses delivered in rapid succession.

Recoil: The bouncing or springing back of an object when it strikes another object.

Tone: The normal degree of nerve tension.

Thrust: The act of putting a bony segment in motion using a directional force.

Toggle: A mechanical principle wherein two levers are hinged at an elbow giving mechanical advantage. Combinations of toggles may be used to multiply or strengthen mechanical advantage.

Toggle Recoil with Torque: A method of using the toggle with rotation (twist) as the toggle straightens, causing the adjusting contact to travel in a spiral path.

Torque: A rotational or twisting vector applied when adjusting certain vertebral subluxations.

Velocity: The speed with which a thrust is delivered.

Conclusion

Considerable evidence substantiates the adjustment being administered for the purpose of correction of vertebral subluxation.[1-11] Studies regarding the different modes[4, 12-86] compare low force methods to those employing a high velocity thrust without recoil, and low velocity vectored force without recoil, high velocity thrust with recoil, low velocity thrust with and without recoil, manually and mechanically assisted thrusts, blocking techniques, and sustained force. These studies are often presented in the context of effects on various physical and physiological parameters.

Although providing useful information, the majority of these studies are limited by uncontrolled variables and lack of statistical power. They do, however, demonstrate that the application of various modes of adjustive care is accompanied by measurable changes in physical and physiological phenomena. The importance of this information, in terms of its linkage to processes used by the body in the correction of subluxation, will be assessed through continued research.

These guidelines consider[86] the modes of adjustive care in common usage, which adhere to one or more of the descriptive terms presented in this chapter, as appropriate for correction of subluxation. However, studies regarding their theoretical basis and efficacy are often conducted by advocates of (those practicing or instructing) the respective techniques. While the information attained in the numerous investigations is not in question, since many of the studies have not passed the scrutiny of peer and editorial review, it is suggested that the advocates of particular modes of adjustive care encourage research by chiropractic colleges, independent universities and other facilities to extend the level of credibility already achieved.

Continuing research and reliability studies are necessary to better understand and refine the underlying mechanisms of action common to the various modes of adjustive care. In addition, it is suggested that more observational and patient self-reporting studies be conducted which deal with quality of life assessments and overall "wellness," to demonstrate the pattern of health benefits which heretofore have been the purview of the patient and the practitioner. A conference sponsored by U.S. Department of Health and Human Services, Public Health Service Agency for Health Care Policy and Research, proposed many different approaches for studying the effects of treatments for which there is no direct evidence of health outcomes.[87]

The CCP recognizes that many subluxation-based chiropractors do not adhere, in totality, to the current hypothetical model thus far described. These practitioners consider two additional components. One is interference with the transmission of nonsynaptic neurological information which is homologous to the Palmer concept of mental impulse. The other limits the misalignment component of the subluxation to the vertebrae and their immediate articulations. While these practitioners may adhere to some concepts of other subluxation models, their practice objectives are based on correction of the vertebral subluxation as proposed by Palmer, which has recently been elaborated by Boone and Dobson.[88-90]

References

1. Fracenboud R. A survey of anterior thoracic adjustments. J Chiro Research 1988; 1:89-92.

2. Gitelman R. 'A chiropractic approach to biomechanical disorders of the lumbar spine and pelvis. Book Excerpt 1979; 297-330.

3. Jessen A. The sacroiliac subluxation. ACA J Chiro 1973; 7(9):865-872.

4. Kale M. How the toggle is used in adjusting. Today's Chiro 1989; 18(4):54-58.

5. Keating J. Technique system application: The Gonstead approach. J Chiropractic Tech 1991; 3(3):135-136.

6. Malik D, Slack J, Wald L, Brooks S. Effectiveness of chiropractic adjustment and physical therapy to treat spinal subluxation. PC Northern J Clin Chiro 1985; 3(2):25-29.

7. McDowall D. The subluxation specific, the adjustment: An early theory of muscle imbalance. ACA J Chiro 1983; 13(1):27-29.

8. Mears D. Adjustment of subluxation as analyzed on lateral cervical x-rays. Digest Chiro Econ 1972; 14(6)14-15.

9. Mears D. Analysis and adjustment of the occiput and cervical spine. Digest Chiro Econ 1970; 12(4):52-53.

10. Nansel D, Cremata E, Carlson J, Szlazak M. Effect of unilateral spinal adjustments on goniometrically-assessed cervical lateral-flexion end-range asymmetrics in otherwise asymptomatic subjects. J Manipulative Physiol Ther 1989; 12(6):419-427.

11. Sandoz R. Some critical reflections on subluxations and adjustments. Ann Swiss Chiro Assoc 1989; 3:7-29.

12. Bryner P. Technique system application: The Gonstead approach. J Chiro Tech 1991; 3(3):134.

13. Decosta A. The correction of lumbosacral and sacroiliac disrelationships. Digest Chiro Econ 1983; 26(3):14-19, 140-143.

14. Fuhr A, Smith D. Accuracy of piezoelectric accelerometers measuring displacement of a spinal adjusting instrument. J Manip Physiol Ther 1986; 9(1):15-21.

15. Gemmell H, Jacobson B, Heng B. Effectiveness of Toftness sacral apex adjustment in correcting fixation of the sacroiliac joint: Preliminary report. Am J Chiro Med 1990; 3(1):5-8.

16.   Gregory R. A kinesiological basis for the C1 adjustment (part 2). Digest Chiro Econ 1983; 25(5):41-44.

17.   Gregory R. A kinesiological basis for the C1 adjustment (part 1). Digest Chiro Econ 1983; 25(4):22-27.

18.   Richards G, Thompson J, Osterbauer P, Fuhr A. Use of pre- and post-CT scans and clinical findings to monitor low force chiropractic care of patients with sciatic neuropathy and lumbar disc herniation: A review. J Manipulative Physiol Ther 1990; 13(1):58.

19.   Terrett A, Webb M. Vertebrobasilar accidents (VA) following cervical spine adjustment manipulation. J Aust Chiro Assoc 1982; 12(50):24-27.

20.   Ungerank R. Implementing the U.S.L.F. technique. Today's Chiro 1989; 18(4):50-52.

21.   Hospers, L. EEG and CEEG studies before and after upper cervical or SOT category II adjustment in children after head trauma, in epilepsy and in "hyperactivity." Proc of the Int'l Conf on Spinal Manip 1992; 84-139.

22.   Insignia, F. A comparative study of activator methods and sacro-occipital technique in low back pain: Short term effects on biomechanical measures. Proc of the Int'l Conf on Spinal Manip 1991; 87-89.

23.   Maltezopoulos V, Armitage N. A comparison of four chiropractic systems in the diagnosis of sacroiliac malfunction. Eur J Chiro 1984; 32(1):4-42.

24.   Unger, J. Precision block placement indicator. Am Chiro 1991; 13(3):8-11.

25.   Unger, J. Short lever manual force mechanically-assisted procedures in sacro occipital technique (SOT). Transactions of the Consortium for Chiropractic Research 1991; 305-309.

26.   Plaugher G, Cremata E, Phillips R. A retrospective consecutive case analysis of pretreatment and comparative static radiological parameters following chiropractic adjustments. J Manipulative Physiol Ther 1990; 13(9):498-506.

27.   Whittingham W, Ellis W, Molyneux T. The effects of manipulation (toggle recoil technique) for headaches with upper cervical joint dysfunction: A pilot study. J Chiro 1994; 17(6):369-375.

28.   Hospers LA, Sweat RW, Hus L, et al. Response of a three year old epileptic child to upper cervical adjustment. Today's Chiro 1987; 15(16):69-76.

29.   Hospers LA, Zozula L, Sweat M. Life upper cervical adjustment in a hyperactive teenager. Today's Chiro 1987; 16(16):73-76.

30.   Bednar, D. Anterior spinal adjustment in inversion traction and effects on the spine. Am Chiro 1991; 13(3):21-24.

31.   Haas, M. The physics of spinal manipulation. Part IV. A theoretical consideration of the physician impact force and energy requirements needed to produce synovial joint cavitation. J Manipulative Physiol Ther 1990; 13(7):378-383.

32. Hessell B, Herzog W, McEwen M, et al. Experimental measurement of the force exerted during spinal manipulation using the Thompson technique. J Manipulative Physiol Ther 1990; 13(8):448-453.

33. Kawchuk G, Herzog W. Biomechanical characterization (fingerprinting) of five novel methods of cervical spine manipulation. J Manipulative Physiol Ther 1993; 16(9):573-577.

34. Osterbauer P, Fuhr A, Hildebrandt R. Mechanical force, manually assisted short lever chiropractic adjustment. J Manipulative Physiol Ther 1992; 15:309-317.

35. Rosen, M. Short lever specific contact procedures. Transactions of the Consortium for Chiropractic Research 1991; 261-264.

36. Gal J, Herzog W, Kawchuk G, et al. Relative movements of vertebral bodies that accompany cracking sounds (cavitation) during manipulative thrusts to unembalmed post-rigor human cadavers. Proc of the Int'l Conf on Spinal Manip 1994; 55.

37. Good, C. An analysis of diversified (lege artis) type adjustments based upon the assisted-resisted model of intervertebral motion unit prestress. Chiro Tech 1992; 4(4):117-123.

38. Greenman P. Principles of manipulation of the cervical spine. J Manual Medicine 1991; 6(3):106-113.

39. Smith D, Fuhr A, Davis B. Skin accelerometer displacement and relative bone movement of adjacent vertebrae in response to chiropractic percussion thrusts. J Manipulative Physiol Ther 1989; 12(1):26-37.

40. Triano J. Modeling of thoracic manipulation: A case study of applied biomechanics. Proc of the Int'l Conf on Spinal Manip 1989; 70-74.

41. Cooperstein R. Thompson technique. Chiropractic Technique 1995; 7(2):60-63.

42. Fracenbound R. A survey of anterior thoracic adjustments. J Chiro Res 1988; 1:89-92.

43. Gemmell H, Jacobson B, Heng B. Effectiveness of Toftness sacral apex adjustment in correcting fixation of the sacroiliac joint: Preliminary Report. Am J Chiro Med 1990; 3(1):5-8.

44. Goodheart G. The cervical challenge. Digest Chiro Econ 1972; 15(2):36-39.

45. Malik D, Slack J, Wald L, et al. Effectiveness of chiropractic adjustment and physical therapy to treat spinal subluxation. PC Northern J Clin Chiro 1985; 3(2):25-29.

46. Mears D. Analysis and adjustment of the occiput and cervical spine. Digest Chiro Econ 1970; 12(4):52-53.

47. Moses D. 1991 year-end compendium. Studies on Logan Basic Piriformis Contact. ACA J Chiro 1991; 28(12):35-37.

48. Nansel D, Cremata E, Carlson J, et al. Effect of unilateral spinal adjustments on goniometrically-assessed cervical lateral-flexion end-range asymmetries in otherwise asymptomatic subjects. J Manipulative Physiol Ther 1989; 12(6):419-427.

49. Richards G, Thompson J, Osterbauer P, et al. Use of pre-and post CT scans and clinical findings to monitor low force chiropractic care of patients with sciatic neuropathy and lumbar disc herniation: A review. J Manipulative Physiol Ther 1990; 13(1):58.

50. Sandoz R. Some critical reflections on subluxations and adjustments. Ann Swiss Chiro Assoc 1989; 3:7-29.

51. Stonebrink R. Thoraco-costal adjustments and related supine techniques. ACA J Chiro 1977; 12(5):855-861.

52. Terrett A, Webb M. Vertebrobasilar accidents (VA) following cervical spine adjustment manipulation. J Aust Chiro Assoc 1982; 12(50):24-27.

53. Boesler D, Warner M, Alpers A, Finnerty EP, Kilmore MA. Efficacy of high-velocity low-amplitude manipulative technique in subjects with low-back pain during menstrual cramping. J Am Osteopath Assoc 1993; 93:203-214.

54. Cassidy JD, Thiel HW, Kirkaldy-Willis WH. Side posture manipulation for lumbar intervertebral disk herniation. J Manipulative Physiol Ther 1993; 16:96-103.

55. Epstein D. Network spinal analysis: A system of health care delivery within the subluxation-based chiropractic model. Journal of Vertebral Subluxation Research, 1996; 1(1):3.

56. Cox JM. Managing low back pain cases with distraction adjustment procedures. Today's Chiro 1993; 22:48-54.

57. Turchin C. Light force techniques for children: An introduction to gentle adjusting techniques for the lower extremity. ICA Review 1993; 49:21-27.

58. Bergmann TF. Various forms of chiropractic technique. Chiropractic Technique 1993; 5:53-55.

59. Bergmann TF. Short lever, specific contact articular chiropractic technique. J Manipulative Physiol Ther 1992; 15:591-595.

60. Triano JJ. Studies on the biomechanical effect of a spinal adjustment. J Manipulative Physiol Ther 1992; 15:71-75.

61. Bergmann TB, Peterson DH, Lawrence DJ. Chiropractic Technique. New York, Churchill Livingstone 1993; 127-128.

62. Cremata EE, Plaugher G, Cox WA. Technique system application: The Gonstead approach. Chiropractic Technique 1991; 3:19-25.

63. Good C. An analysis of diversified (lege artis) type adjustments upon the assisted-resisted model of intervertebral motion unit prestress. Chiropractic Technique 1992; 4:117-123.

64. Evans DP, Burke MS, Lloyd KN, et al. Lumbar spinal manipulation on trial: 1. Clinical assessment. Rheum Rehabil 1978; 17:46-53.

65. Tran TA, Kirby JD. The effectiveness of upper cervical adjustment upon the normal physiology of the heart. ACA J Chiro 1977; XIS:58-62.

66. Briggs L, Boone WR. Effects of a chiropractic adjustment on changes in pupillary diameter: A model for evaluating somatovisceral response. J Manipulative Physiol Ther 1988; 11:181-189.

67. Palmer DD. The chiropractor's adjuster, the science, art and philosophy of chiropractic. Portland, Ore. Portland Printing House, 1910.

68. VanRumpt R. Directional non-force technique notes. Beverly Hills, Calif, Directional Non-Force Technique, 1987.

69. Osterbauer PJ, Fuhr AW. The current status of activator methods chiropractic technique, theory, and training. Chiropractic Technique 1990; 2:168.

70. Bartol KM. A model for the categorization of chiropractic treatment procedures. Chiropractic Technique 1991; 3:78.

71. Kaminski M, Boal R, Gillette RG, et al. A model for the evaluation of chiropractic methods. J Manipulative Physiol Ther 1987; 10:61.

72. Kaminski M. Evaluation of chiropractic methods. Chiropractic Technique 1990; 2:3.

73. Osterbauer PJ, Fuhr AW, Hildebrandt RW. Mechanical force manually adjusted short lever chiropractic adjustment. J Manipulative Physiol Ther 1992; 15:309-317.

74. Smith DB, Fuhr AW, Davis BP. Skin accelerometer displacement and relative bone movement of adjacent vertebrae in response to chiropractic percussion thrusts. J Manipulative Physiol Ther 1989; 12:26-37.

75. Triano JJ. The biomechanics of the chiropractic adjustment. J Manipulative Physiol Ther 1992; 15:71-75.

76. Van Rumpt R. Directional non-force technique notes. In Directional Non-Force Technique. Beverly Hills, Calif, 1987.

77. Thompson C. Technique Reference Manual. Thompson Educational Workshops. Ill, SM & Williams Manufacturing, 1987.

78. Nansel DD, Waldorf The, Cooperstein R. Effect of cervical spinal adjustments on lumbar paraspinal muscle tone: Evidence for facilitation of intersegmental tonic neck reflexes. J Manipulative Physiol Ther 1993; 16:91-95.

79. Hessel BW, Herzog W, Conway PIW, et al. Experimental measurement of the force exerted during spinal manipulation using the Thompson technique. J. Manipulative Physiol Ther 1990; 13:448-453.

80. Herzog W. Biomechanical studies of spinal manipulative therapy. J Can Chiro Assoc 1991; 35:156-164.

81. Kawchuk GN, Herzog W, Hasleer EM. Forces generated during spinal manipulative therapy of the cervical spine. J Manipulative Physiol Ther 1992; 15:275-278.

82. Gal JM, Herzog W, Kawchuk G, et al. Movements of vertebrae during PA adjustment to unembalmed cadavers. Proceedings of the 1993 International Conference on Spinal Manipulation, Montreal, Foundation of Chiropractic Education and Research, 1993; 15.

83. Herzog W, Gal J, Conway P, et al. Vertebral movement during spinal manipulative therapy. Proceedings of the 1993 International Conference on Spinal Manipulation, Montreal, Foundation of Chiropractic Education and Research, 1993; 14.

84. Lee M, Svensson NL. Effect of loading frequency response of the spine to lumbar posteroanterior forces. J Manipulative Physiol Ther 1993; 16:439-446.

85. Wood J, Adams AA, Hansmeter D. Force and time characteristics of Pierce technique cervical adjustments. Chiropractic: J Chiro Research and Clinical Investigation 1994; 9:39-44.

86. Bergmann TF. Chiropractic technique: An overview. Advances in Chiropractic 1995; 2:429-431.

87. Methodology Perspectives. Clinical Practice Guideline Development. US Department of Health and Human Services, Public Health Service, Agency for Health Care Policy and Research, 1994; 5-12.

88. Boone WR, Dobson GJ. A proposed vertebral subluxation model reflecting traditional concepts and recent advances in health and science. Journal of Vertebral Subluxation Research 1996; 1(1) 19-30.

89. Boone WR, Dobson GJ. A proposed vertebral subluxation model reflecting traditional concepts and recent advances in health and science: Part II. Journal of Vertebral Subluxation Research 1996; 1(2):23-30.

90. Boone WR, Dobson GJ. A proposed vertebral subluxation model reflecting traditional concepts and recent advances in health and science: Part III. Journal of Vertebral Subluxation Research 1997; 1(3)25-33.

7 Duration of Care for Correction of Vertebral Subluxation

RECOMMENDATION

Since the duration of care for correction of vertebral subluxation is patient specific, frequency of visits should be based upon the reduction and eventual resolution of indicators of vertebral subluxation. Since neither the scientific nor clinical literature provides any compelling evidence that substantiates or correlates any specific time period for the correction of vertebral subluxation, this recommendation has several components which are expressed as follows:

a) Based on the variety of assessments utilized in the chiropractic profession, the quantity of indicators may vary, thus affecting the periodicity of their appearance and disappearance, which is tantamount to correction of vertebral subluxation.

b) Vertebral subluxation, not being a singular episodic event such as a strain or sprain, may be corrected but reappear, which necessitates careful monitoring and results in a wide variation in the number of adjustments required to affect a longer-term correction.

c) Based on the integrity of the spine in terms of degree and extent of degeneration, the frequency of assessments, and the necessity for corrective adjustments, may vary considerably.

d) Because the duration of care is being considered relative to the correction of vertebral subluxation, it is independent of clinical manifestations of specific dysfunctions, diseases, or syndromes. Treatment protocols and duration of care for these conditions are addressed in other guidelines, which may be appropriate for any practitioner whose clinical interests include alleviation of such conditions.

Rating: Established
Evidence: E, L

Commentary

Attempts have been made to identify an appropriate number and frequency of chiropractic visits based on type of condition and degree of severity.[1-24] Unfortunately, these recommendations are based merely on consensus, and research to support these recommendations is lacking. Moreover, little to no delineation has been made in the duration of care literature base between care for specific symptomatic profiles such as low-back pain, and long-term subluxation-specific care.

Two studies were found which addressed quality of life issues in patients under chiropractic care. One large, well-designed retrospective study assessing patient reported quality of life found no clinical end point where improvement reached a plateau.[25] A second study involved a detailed examination of a database collected during a randomized clinical trial testing the effectiveness of a comprehensive geriatric assessment program. It was reported that compared to non-chiropractic patients, chiropractic patients in this population were less likely to have been hospitalized, less likely to have used a nursing home, more likely to report a better health status, more likely to exercise vigorously, and more likely to be mobile in the community. Furthermore, they were less likely to use prescription drugs.[26]

It is the position of the Guideline Panel that individual differences in each patient and the unique circumstances of each clinical encounter preclude the formulation of "cookbook" recommendations for frequency and duration of care.

The appropriateness of chiropractic care should be determined by objective indicators of vertebral subluxation.

References

1.   Balduc H. How chiropractic care can promote wellness. Northwestern College of Chiropractic, Bloomington, MN.

2.   Coile J, Russel C. "Promoting health," the new medicine: reshaping medical practice and health care management. Aspen Publ, Inc, Rockville, MD 1990; 151-166.

3.   Coulter ID. The patient, the practitioner, and wellness: Paradigm lost, paradigm gained. J Manipulative Physiol Ther 1990; 13(2):107-111.

4.   Flesia JM (President, Renaissance International and President, Chiropractic Basic Science Research Foundation). Vertebral subluxation degeneration complex, a review of therapeutic necessity for FSC well patient care, in: Seminar Notes (The New Renaissance, "Global Chiropractic ... one patient at a time"), 7-36, including the 496 various papers, referenced therein.

5.   Hildebrandt R. Chiropractic physicians as members of the health care delivery system: The case for increased utilization. J Manipulative Physiol Ther 1980; 3(1):23-32.

6.   Jamison J. Chiropractic as conventional health care. J Aust Chiro Assoc 1989; 15(2):55-59.

7.   Jamison J. Preventive chiropractic and the chiropractic management of visceral conditions: Is the cost to chiropractic acceptance justified by the benefits to health care? J Aust Chiro Asso 1991; 9(3):95-101.

8.   Vear H. The role of chiropractic in preventive health care. J Can Chiro Assoc 1974; 18(4):10-3.

9.   Olson RE. Chiropractic/physical therapy treatment standards: a reference guide. Data Management Ventures, Inc. Atlanta, GA, 1987.

10.   Lang MG (chm) et al. Oregon chiropractic practices and utilization guidelines for neuromusculoskeletal conditions. Oregon Chiropractic Practice and Utilization Guidelines Committee.

11.   Minnesota Chiropractic Association. Standards of practice. Roseville, MN, 1991.

12.   Ohio State Chiropractic Association. The chiropractic manual for insurance personnel. Columbus, Ohio, 1988-1990.

13.   Hansen DT (ed). Chiropractic standards and utilization guidelines in the care and treatment of injured workers. Chiropractic Advisory Committee, Department of Labor and Industries, State of Washington, 1988.

14.   Leblanc F (ed). Scientific approach to the assessment and management of activity-related spinal disorders. Spine 1987; 12:16-21.

15. Haldeman S. Presidential address, North American Spine Society: Failure of the pathology model to predict back pain. Spine 1990; 15:718-24.

16. Frymoyer J. Back pain and sciatica. N Engl J Med 1988; 318:291-300.

17. Mayer T, Gatchel R. Functional restoration for spinal disorders: A sports medicine approach. Philadelphia, Lea & Febiger, 1988.

18. Bronfort G. Chiropractic treatment of low-back pain: a prospective survey. J Manipulative Physiol Ther 1986; 9:99-133.

19. Phillips RB, Butler R. Survey of chiropractic in Dade County, Florida. J Manipulative Physiol Ther 1982; 5:83-9.

20. Phillips R. A survey of Utah chiropractic patients. ACA J Chiro 1981; 18:113-28.

21. Guifu C, Zongmin L, Zhenzhong You, Jiaghua W. Lateral rotatory manipulative maneuver in the treatment of subluxation and synovial entrapment of lumbar facet joints. The Trad Chin Med 1984; 4:211-12.

22. Jarvis KB, Phillips RB, Morris EK. Cost per case comparison of back injury claims of chiropractic versus medical management for conditions with identical diagnostic codes. J Occup Med 1991; 33:847-52.

23, Sullivan MD, Turner JA, Romano J. Chronic pain in primary care identification and management of psychosocial factors. J Fam Pract 1991; 32:193-199.

24. Waddell G, Main CJ, Morris EW, DiPaola M, Gray L. Chronic low back pain, psychologic distress and illness behavior. Spine 1984; 9:209-13.

25. Blanks RH, Schuster TL, Dobson M. A retrospective assessment of network care using a survey of self-rated health, wellness, and quality of life. Journal of Vertebral Subluxation Research 1997; 1(4):15-31.

26. Coulter I, Hurwitz E, Aronow H, Cassata D, Beck J. Chiropractic patients in a comprehensive home-based geriatric assessment, follow-up and health promotion program. Topics in Clinical Chiropractic 1996; 3(2):46-55.

8 Chiropractic Care of Children

RECOMMENDATION

Since vertebral subluxation may affect individuals at any age, chiropractic care may be indicated at any time after birth. As with any age group, however, care must be taken to select adjustment methods most appropriate to the patient's stage of development and overall spinal integrity. Parental education by the subluxation-centered chiropractor concerning the importance of evaluating children for the presence of vertebral subluxation is encouraged.

Rating: Established

Evidence: E, L

Commentary

Schneier and Burns[1] published the results of a blinded study describing the relationship of atlanto-occipital hypermobility to sudden infant death syndrome (SIDS). These authors described the phenomenon of "atlas inversion" where the posterior arch of C-1 enters the foramen magnum. They further stated, "Relative measurements suggested that a correlation existed between instability in the atlanto-occipital articulation and sudden infant death syndrome." Instability is a manifestation of vertebral subluxation.

These findings corroborate those of Gilles, Bina and Sotrel in their paper, "Infantile atlanto-occipital instability."[2] These investigators studied 17 infant cadavers. Eleven were SIDS cases and six were non-SIDS cases. Ten of the 17 cases demonstrated atlas inversion, and all ten cases were in the SIDS group. These authors also suggested that atlanto-occipital instability may be a factor in other conditions. They stated, "At this early stage in the development of our notions about the potential contribution of atlanto-occipital instability to deaths in infants, it is very difficult to assess the role of this proposed mechanism in the death of an infant with a conventional disease. Thus, one might anticipate that the 'controls' will be contaminated by children who had a conventional disease, but whose death was, in fact, caused by this mechanism."

Towbin[3] addressed the clinical significance of spinal cord and brain stem injury at birth, noting that such damage is often latent and undiagnosed. According to Towbin, "Death of the fetus may occur during delivery or, with respiratory function depressed, a short period after birth. Infants who survive the initial effects may be left with severe nervous system defects. In some, the neurologic sequellae are attributable directly to the primary lesion in the cord or brain stem; in others, secondary cerebral damage results, a consequence of the imposed period of hypoxia at birth." Chesire[4] described three cases of traumatic myelopathy in children without demonstrable vertebral trauma. In this paper, the classical mechanism of trauma is said to be hyperextension of the cervical spine in a difficult breech delivery. Although tetraplegia may result, the x-rays are described as "usually normal."

Complicated deliveries represent a higher risk to the child of suffering spinal cord damage during the birth process. High cervical spinal cord injury in neonates is a specific complication of forceps rotation. The vacuum extractor exerts considerable traction force. Fetal skull fracture can result, and its true incidence may be higher than expected, considering that few neonates with normal neurologic behavior undergo skull x-ray.[5-7] Byers[8] published an excellent review paper addressing spinal cord damage during the birth process. Traction and rotational stresses applied to the spinal axis were listed as causes of spinal cord injury during birth.

The vagus nerve is involved in mechanisms associated with control of tidal volume, breathing rate, and respiratory reflexes. Sachis et al.[9] performed histological examinations of the vagus nerve in infants who died of SIDS and those who died of other conditions. Significant differences were noted between the two groups. Several hypotheses were proposed by authors to explain the data, including damage to the vagus nerve resulting in delayed development.

Gutman[10] described how "relational disturbance" between occiput and atlas can lead to "blocked atlantal nerve syndrome" in children and adults. The author listed a variety of conditions which appear clinically related to this syndrome. Although SIDS was not discussed as an entity, the author stated that a brain stem component is a part of this syndrome. It was concluded that for those affected, "manual treatment" by a qualified practitioner is appropriate.

In her paper "Physical stresses of childhood that could lead to need for chiropractic care," presented at the first National Conference on Chiropractic and Pediatrics, McMullen[11] stated, "Any condition that arises to change the normal birth process... frequently results in subluxation at the level of greatest stress. Severe subluxation resulting in nerve damage may be clinically obvious at birth (e.g., Bell's, Erb's and Klumpke's palsies), however, more frequently the trauma remains subclinical with symptoms arising at a later time. These symptoms include, but are not limited to, irritability, colic, failure-to-thrive syndromes, and those syndromes associated with lowered immune responses. These subluxations should be analyzed and corrected as soon as possible after birth to prevent these associated conditions."

Bonci and Wynne[12] and Stiga[13] published papers discussing the relationship between chiropractic theory and SIDS etiology. Banks et al.[14] stated "Functional disturbances in the brainstem and cervical spinal cord areas related to the neurophysiology of respiration may contribute the clinical factors associated with sudden infant death syndrome...Any process, whether genetic, biochemical, biomechanical or traumatic, that alters normal development of the respiratory control centers related to spinal constriction and compression following birth trauma may be contributory to sudden infant death syndrome."

Other traumatic events of childhood may produce vertebral subluxations. Orenstein et al.[15] did a retrospective chart review involving 73 children who presented at a children's hospital with cervical spine injuries. Sixty-seven percent of these injuries were traffic related resulting from motor-vehicle crashes. The injured children were passengers in an automobile, pedestrians, or bicyclists. The mean age of the patients surveyed was 8.6 years, with bimodal peaks at 2 to 4 and 12 to 15 years. The authors noted that younger children sustained more severe injuries than older children. Distraction and subluxation injuries were the most common injuries in children aged 8 years and younger. Fractures were more common in older children.

Glass et al.[16] evaluated 35 children with lumbar spine injuries following blunt trauma. Thirty-one of these children were injured in motor-vehicle crashes. Abnormalities noted on plain radiographs and CT scans included subluxation, distraction, and fracture alone or in combination. The authors stated, "Children involved in motor-vehicle crashes are at a high risk for lumbar spine injuries... Lumbar spine radiographs are necessary in all cases with suspected lumbar spine injury..." This paper underscores the need to evaluate the entire spine in cases of motor-vehicle accidents, not just the cervical region. It may be cited when claims for lumbar radiographs are questioned in cases of children involved in car accidents.

Rachesky et al.[17] reported that on the cervical spine radiographs of children under 18 they examined, vehicular accidents accounted for 36% of radiographic abnormalities. It was further stated that clinical assessment of a complaint of neck pain or involvement in a vehicular accident with head trauma would have identified all cases of cervical spine injury.

Other authors have described aspects of cervical spine injuries in children involved in motor-vehicle accidents. Hill et al.[18] noted that 31% of the pediatric neck injuries reviewed were the result of motor-vehicle accidents. In younger children (under 8 years of age) subluxation was seen more frequently than fracture. Agran[19] stated that non-crash vehicular events may cause injuries to children. Non-crash events discussed in this paper included sudden stops, swerves, turns, and movement of unrestrained children in the vehicle.

Roberts et al.[20] described a case where a child involved in a motor-vehicle accident sustained a "whiplash" injury resulting in immediate neck and back pain. Neurobehavioral abnormalities increased in the two-year period following the accident. Four years after the accident, symptoms persisted. Position emission tomography (PET scan) demonstrated evidence of brain dysfunction.

The clinical manifestations of pediatric cervical spine injury may be diverse. Biedermann[21] stated that a wide range of pediatric symptomatology may result from suboccipital strain. The disorders reported include fever of unknown origin, loss of appetite, sleeping disorders, asymmetric motor patterns, and alterations of posture. Maigne[22] stated that trauma to the cervical spine and head can cause such problems as headaches, vestibular troubles, auditory problems and psychic disturbances. Gutmann[23] discussed the diverse array of signs and symptoms which can occur as a result of biomechanical dysfunction in the cervical spine. Others have also reported various pathoneurophysiological changes in children,[24-31] as well as reduction of pathology following chiropractic care.[29,31-41,44] In the chiropractic literature, Clow[42] published a paper addressing pediatric cervical acceleration/deceleration injuries.

Two peer reviewed journals, Chiropractic Pediatrics and the Journal of Clinical Chiropractic Pediatrics are being published to disseminate critically reviewed papers in this field. Additionally, courses in pediatrics are offered at the professional and postgraduate levels at accredited chiropractic colleges and by the International Chiropractic Pediatric Association.

The pediatric case history and physical examination necessarily differ in content and scope from those of adult patients. Even taking into consideration the difference between the two populations, however, a recent quasi meta-analysis reveals an extremely low risk for chiropractic pediatric patients receiving adjustments.[43]

References

1. Schneier M, Burns RE: Atlanto-occipital hypermobility in sudden infant death syndrome. Chiropractic: J Chiro Research and Clinical Investigation 1991; 7(2):33.

2. Gilles FH, Bina M, Sotrel A. Infantile atlanto-occipital instability. Am J Dis Child 1979; 133:30.

3. Towbin A. Latent spinal cord and brain stem injury in newborn infants. Develop Med Child Neurol 1969; 11:54.

4. Chesire DJE. The paediatric syndrome of traumatic myelopathy without demonstrable vertebral injury. Paraplegia 1977-78; 15:74.

5. Menticoglou SM, Peerlman M, Manning FA. High cervical spinal cord injury in neonates delivered with forceps; report of 15 cases. Obstet Gynecol 1995; 86(4 Pt 1):589-94.

6. Hickey K, McKenna P. Skull fracture caused by vacuum extraction. Obstet Gynecol 1996; 88(4 Pt. 2):671.

7. Ross MG. Skull fracture caused by vacuum extraction. Obstet Gynecol 1997; 89(2):319.

8. Byers RK. Spinal-cord injuries during birth. Develop Med Child Neurol 1975 17(1):103.

9. Sachis PN, Armstrong DL, Becker LE, Bryan AC. The vagus nerve and sudden infant death syndrome: a morphometric study. J Pediatrics 1981 98(2):278.

10. Gutman G. Blocked atlantal nerve syndrome in infants and small children. Originally published in Manuelle Medizin, Springer-Verlag, 1987. English translation published in International Review of Chiropractic 1990 46(4):37.

11. McMullen M. Physical stresses of childhood that could lead to need for chiropractic care. Proceedings of the National Conference on Chiropractic and Pediatrics. Arlington, VA: International Chiropractors Association, 1991.

12. Bonci A, Wynne C. The interface between sudden infant death syndrome and chiropractic. Journal of Chiropractic Research 1989; 5(3):78.

13. Stiga J: Sudden infant death syndrome. American Chiropractor 1983:28.

14. Banks B, Beck R, Columbus M, et al. Sudden infant death syndrome: a literature review with chiropractic implications. J Manipulative Physiol Ther 1987; 10(5):246.

15. Orenstein JB, Klein BL, Gotschall CS, et al. Age and outcome in pediatric cervical spine injury: 11-year experience. Pediatr Emerg Care 1994; 10(3):132.

16. Glass RB, Sivit CJ, Sturm PF, et al, Lumbar spine injury in a pediatric population: difficulties with computed tomographic diagnosis. J Trauma 1994; 37(5):815.

17. Racheskey I, Boyce WT, Duncan B, et al. Clinical prediction of cervical spine injuries in children. Radiographic abnormalities. Am J Dis Child 1987; 141(2):199.

18. Hill SA, Miller CA, Kosnik EJ, Hunt WE. Pediatric neck injuries. A clinical study. J Neurosurg 1984; 60(4):700.

19. Agran PF. Motor vehicle occupant injuries in noncrash events. Pediatrics 1981; 67(6):838.

20. Roberts MA, Manshadi FF, Bushnell DL, Hines ME. Neurobehavioral dysfunction following mild traumatic brain injury in childhood: a case report with positive findings on positron emission tomography (PET). Brain Inj 1995; 9(5):427.

21. Biedermann H. Kinematic imbalances due to suboccipital strain in newborns. Manual Medicine 1992; 6:151.

22. Maigne R. Orthopedic medicine, a new approach to vertebral manipulations. Charles C. Thomas, 1972.

23. Gutmann G. Blocked atlantal nerve syndrome in infants and small children. ICA Review 1990; 46(4):37.

24. Abroms IF, Bresnan MJ, Zuckerman JE, Fischer EG, Strand R. Cervical cord injuries secondary to hyperextension of the head in breech presentations. Obstet Gynecol 1973; 41(3):369-378.

25. Glasauer FE, Cares HL. Biomechanical features of traumatic paraplegia in infancy. J of Trauma 1973; 3(2):166-170.

26. Okumura H, Homma TT. Juvenile compression myelopathy in the cervical spine. Spine 1994; 19(1):72-76.

27. Lanska MJ, Roessmann R, Wiznitzer M. Magnetic resonance imaging in cervical cord birth injury. Pediatrics 1990; 85(5):760-764.

28. Ono K, et al. Atlantoaxial rotatory fixation: radiographic study of its mechanism. Spine 1985; 10(7):602-608.

29. Harris SL, Wood KW. Resolution of infantile Erb's palsy utilizing chiropractic treatment. J Manipulative Physiol Ther 1993; 16(6):415-418.

30. BenEliyahu DJ. The detection and management of pediatric whiplash injuries. Proceedings of the National Conference on Chiropractic & Pediatrics October 1993; Palm Springs, ICA publisher, 53-57.

31. Araghi H. Post-traumatic evaluation and treatment of the pediatric patient with head injury: a case report. Proceedings of the National Conference of Chiropractic & Pediatrics. November 1992; ICA publisher. Colorado Springs 1-8.

32. Peet P. Child with chronic illness: respiratory infections, ADHD, and fatigue. Response to chiropractic care. Chiropractic Pediatrics 1997; 3(1):12.

33. Reed WR, et al. Chiropractic management of primary nocturnal enuretic children. In: Proceedings of the 3rd National Conference of Chiropractic and Pediatrics. Arlington, VA: ICA publisher 1993:64-82.

34. Hudgkins DJ, et al. Evaluation and chiropractic treatment of the pediatric patient with nocturnal enuresis: a case report. In: Proceedings of thyromegaly 4th National Conference on Chiropractic and Pediatrics. Arlington, VA. ICA publisher 1994:80-84.

35. Bachman T, Lantz CA. Management of pediatric asthma and enuresis with probable traumatic etiology. In: Proceedings of the 1st National Conference on Chiropractic and Pediatrics, Arlington, VA: ICA publisher 1991:14-22.

36. Nilsson N, Christiansen B. Prognostic factors in bronchial asthma in chiropractic practice. J Aust Chiro Assoc 1988; 18(3):85-87.

37. Vernon LF, Vernon G. A scientific hypothesis for the efficacy of chiropractic manipulation in the pediatric asthmatic patient. Chiropractic Pediatrics 1995; 1(4):7-8.

38. Langley C. Epileptic seizures, nocturnal enuresis, ADD. Chiropractic Pediatrics 1994; 1(1):21-22.

39. Klougart N, et al. Infantile colic treated by chiropractors: a prospective study of 316 cases. J Manip Physiol Ther 1989; 12(4):281-288.

40. Nilsson N. Infant colic and chiropractic. Eur J Chir 1985; 33(4):264-265.

41. Graham RL, Pistolese RA. An impairment rating analysis of asthmatic children under chiropractic care. Journal of Vertebral Subluxation Research 1997; 1(4):41-48.

42. Clow BJE: Pediatric cervical acceleration/deceleration injuries. Journal of Clinical Chiropractic Pediatrics 1996; 1(1):36.

43. Pistolese RA. Risk assessment of neurological and/or vertebrobasilar complications in the pediatric chiropractic patient. Journal of Vertebral Subluxation Research 1998; 2(2):In press.

44. Blum K, Holder JM. Attention deficit disorders (ADD). Biogenic aspects. Chiropractic Pediatrics 1994; 1(2):21-23.

9 Patient Safety

RECOMMENDATION

Patient safety encompasses the entire spectrum of care offered by the chiropractor. Consequently, it is important to define at the onset, the nature of the practice as well as the limits of care to be offered. Minimally this should include a "Terms of Acceptance" document between the practitioner and the patient. Additionally, all aspects of clinical practice should be carefully chosen to offer the patient the greatest advantage with the minimum of risk.
Rating: Established
Evidence: E, L

Commentary

Patient safety is assured by more than the practitioner's causing no harm. Since every consumer of health care is ultimately responsible for his/her own health choices, patient safety is also a matter of the availability of accurate and adequate information with which the patient must make these choices. The patient's expectations should be consistent with the provider's goals. If the patient perceives those goals as anything different, proper and safe choices cannot be assured. Thus, it is important to recognize that chiropractic is a limited, primary profession which contributes to health by addressing the safe detection, location, and correction or stabilization of vertebral subluxation(s). It is important that the chiropractor take the steps necessary to foster proper patient perception and expectation of the practitioner's professional goals and responsibilities. It is within this context that patient safety is addressed in this chapter.

A "Terms of Acceptance" is the recorded written informed consent agreement between a chiropractor and the patient. This document provides the patient with disclosure of the responsibilities of the chiropractor and limits of chiropractic, and the reasonable benefit to be expected. This enables the patient to make an informed choice either to engage the services of the chiropractor, aware of the intended purpose of the care involved, or not to engage those services if the proposed goals are not acceptable or not desired. This embodies the responsibility of assuring patient safety by not providing false or misleading promises, claims or pretenses to the patient.[1-7]

Professional Referral: Professional referral requires authority and competence to acquire accurate information concerning matters within the scope and practice of the professional to whom a referral is made. There are two types of professional referrals made by chiropractors:

(A) **Intraprofessional referral:** Chiropractors, by virtue of their professional objective, education, and experience, have authority and competence to make direct referrals within the scope and practice of chiropractic. Such a referral may be made when the attending chiropractor is not able to address the specific chiropractic needs of a particular patient. Under these circumstances, the chiropractor may refer the patient directly to or consult with another chiropractor better suited by skill, experience or training to address the patient's chiropractic needs.

(B) **Interprofessional referral:** In the course of patient assessment and the delivery of chiropractic care, a practitioner may encounter findings which are outside his/her professional and/or legal scope, responsibility, or authority to address. The chiropractor has a responsibility to report such findings to the patient, and record their existence. Additionally, the patient should be advised that it is outside the responsibility and scope of chiropractic to offer advice, assessment or significance, diagnosis, prognosis, or treatment for said findings and that, if the patient chooses, he/she may consult with another provider, while continuing to have his/her chiropractic needs addressed.

Rare case reports of adverse events following spinal "manipulation" exist in the literature. However, scientific evidence of a causal relationship between such adverse events and the "manipulation" is lacking. Furthermore, spinal adjustment and spinal manipulation are not synonymous terms.

In the case of strokes purportedly associated with "manipulation," the panel noted significant shortcomings in the literature. A summary of the relevant literature follows:

*Lee[8] attempted to obtain an estimate of how often practicing neurologists in California encountered unexpected strokes, myelopathies, or radiculopathies following "chiropractic manipulation." Neurologists were asked the number of patients evaluated over the preceding two years who suffered a neurological complication within 24 hours of receiving "chiropractic manipulation." Fifty-five strokes were reported. The author stated, "Patients, physicians, and chiropractors should be aware of the risk of neurologic complications associated with chiropractic manipulation." No support was offered to substantiate the premise that a causal relationship existed between the stroke and the event(s) of the preceding 24 hours.

*In a letter to the editor of the Journal of Manipulative and Physiological Therapeutics, Myler[9] wrote, "I was curious how the risk of fatal stroke after cervical manipulation, placed at 0.00025%[10] compared with the risk of (fatal) stroke in the general population of the United States." According to data obtained from the National Center for Health Statistics, the mortality rate from stroke in the general population was calculated to be 0.00057%. If these data are correct, the risk of a fatal stroke following "cervical manipulation" is less than half the risk of fatal stroke in the general population.

*Jaskoviak[11] reported that not a single case of vertebral artery stroke occurred in approximately five million cervical "manipulations" at the National College of Chiropractic Clinic from 1965 to 1980.

*Osteopathic authors Vick, et al.[12] reported that from 1923 to 1993, there were only 185 reports of injury associated with "several million treatments."

*Pistolese[13] has constructed a risk assessment for pediatric chiropractic patients. His findings covering approximately the last 30 years indicate a risk of a neurological and/or vertebrobasilar accident during a chiropractic visit about one in every 250,000,000 visits.

*An article in the "Back Letter"[14] noted that "In scientific terms, all these figures are rough guesses at best... There is currently no accurate data on the total number of cervical manipulations performed every year or the total number of complications. Both figures would be necessary to arrive at an accurate estimate. In addition, none of the studies in the medical literature adequately control for other risk factors and co-morbidities."

*Leboeuf-Yde et al.[15] suggested that there may be an over-reporting of "spinal manipulative therapy" related injuries. The authors reported cases involving two fatal strokes, a heart attack, a bleeding basilar aneurysm, paresis of an arm and a leg, and cauda equina syndrome which occurred in individuals who were considering chiropractic care, yet because of chance, did not receive it. Had these events been temporally related to a chiropractic office visit, they may have been inappropriately attributed to chiropractic care.

*In many cases of strokes attributed to chiropractic care, the "operator" was not a chiropractor at all. Terrett[16] observed that "manipulations" administered by Kung Fu practitioner, GPs, osteopaths, physiotherapists, a wife, a blind masseur, and an Indian barber were incorrectly attributed to chiropractors. As Terrett wrote, "The words chiropractic and chiropractor have been incorrectly used in numerous publications dealing with SMT injury by medical authors, respected medical journals and medical organizations. In many cases, this is not accidental; the authors had access to original reports that identified the practitioner involved as a non-chiropractor. The true incidence of such reporting cannot be determined. Such reporting adversely affects the reader's opinion of chiropractic and chiropractors."

*Another error made in these reports was failure to differentiate "cervical manipulation" from specific chiropractic adjustment. Klougart et al.[17] published risk estimates which revealed differences which were dependent upon the type of technique used by the chiropractor.

The panel found no competent evidence that specific chiropractic adjustments cause strokes. Although vertebrobasilar screening procedures are taught in chiropractic colleges, no reliable screening tests were identified which enable a chiropractor to identify patients who are at risk for stroke.

After examining twelve patients with dizziness reproduced by extension rotation and twenty healthy controls with Doppler ultrasound of the vertebral arteries, Cote, et al.[18] concluded, "We were unable to demonstrate that the extension-rotation test is a valid clinical screening procedure to detect decreased blood flow in the vertebral artery. The value of this test for screening patients at risk of stroke after cervical manipulation is questionable." Terrett[19] noted, "There is no evidence which suggests that positive tests have any correlation to future VBS (vertebrobasilar stroke) and SMT (spinal manipulative therapy)." Despite this lack of evidence, some have suggested that failure to employ such tests could place a chiropractor in a less defensible position should litigation ensue following a CVA.[20]

References

1.   Bolton SP. Informed consent revisited. J Aust Chiro Assoc 1990; 20(4):134-138.

2.   Cary P. Informed consent - the new reality. J Can Chiro Assoc 1988; 32(2):91-94.

3.   Gill KM. Efforts to prevent malpractice suits. Princeton Insurance Company, Princeton, NJ, May 4, 1989.

4.   Gotlib A. The nature of the informed consent doctrine and the chiropractor. J Can Chiro Assoc 1984; 28(2):272-274.

5.   Hug PR. General considerations of "consent." J Chiro 1985; 22(12):52-53.

6.   Jackson R, Schafer R. Basic chiropractic paraprofessional manual, Chapter XII. ACA, Des Moines, 1A. XII:3-4, 1978.

7.   White B. Ethical issues surrounding informed consent. Part II. Components of a morally valid consent and conditions that impair its validity. Urol Nurs 1989; 9(4):4-9.

8.   Lee K. Neurologic complications following chiropractic manipulation: a survey of California neurologists. Neurology 1995; 45:1213.

9.   Myler L. Letter to the editor. J Manipulative Physiol Ther 1996;19:357.

10.   Dabbs V, Lauretti WJ. A risk assessment of cervical manipulation vs. NSAIDS for the treatment of neck pain. J Manipulative Physiol Ther 1995; 18:530.

11.   Jaskoviac P. Complications arising from manipulation of the cervical spine. J Manipulative Physiol Ther 1980; 3:213.

12.   Vick D, McKay C, Zengerle C. The safety of manipulative treatment: review of the literature from 1925 to 1993. JAOA 1996; 96:113.

13.   Pistolese RA. Risk assessment of neurological and/or vertebrobasilar complications in the pediatric chiropractic patients. Journal of Vertebral Subluxation Research 1998; 2(2): In·Press.

14.   What about the serious complications of cervical manipulation? The Back Letter 1996; 11:115.

15.   Leboeuf-Yde C, Rasmussen LR, Klougart N. The risk of over-reporting spinal manipulative therapy-induced injuries; a description of some cases that failed to burden the statistics. J Manipulative Physiol Ther 1996; 19:536.

16.   Terrett AGJ. Misuse of the literature by medical authors in discussing spinal manipulative therapy injury. J Manipulative Physiol Ther 1995; 18:203.

17. Klougart N, Leboeuf-Yde C, Rasmussen LR. Safety in chiropractic practice, Part I; The occurrence of cerebrovascular accidents after manipulation to the neck in Denmark from 1978-1988. J Manipulative Physiol Ther 1996; 19:371.

18. Cote P, Kreitz B, Cassidy J, Thiel H. The validity of the extension-rotation test as a clinical screening procedure before neck manipulation: a secondary analysis. J Manipulative Physiol Ther 1996; 19:159.

19. Terrett AGJ. Vertebrobasilar stroke following manipulation. NCMIC, Des Moines, 1996, page 32.

20. Ferezy JS. The Chiropractic Neurological examination. Aspen Publishers. Gaithersburg, MD 1992.

10 Professional Development

RECOMMENDATION

Continuing professional development, as in all responsible health professions, is a necessary component of maintaining a high standard for both the practitioner and the profession. Continuing development should be directed to areas germane to each individual practice, including but not limited to: credentialing, continuing education programs, participation in professional organizations, ethics forums, and legal issues.

Rating: Established
Evidence: E, L

Commentary

Continuing professional development is currently widely mandated by most licensing jurisdictions, or encouraged through most professional organizations. Perhaps the most compelling reason for advocating this type of on-going education is to afford practitioners the opportunity to keep abreast of current issues, techniques, and methods which serve to enhance patient care. The fact that most programs are conducted by individuals skilled in the topics presented, also provides a high ratio of quality information delivered in a relatively short period. Thus, professional development serves not only the practitioner, but ultimately benefits the patient through enhanced practice skills acquired in different areas by the chiropractor.[1-14]

In addition to formal postgraduate education courses, other opportunities for professional development may include:

- Reading scholarly journals
- Attending scientific symposia
- Participation in research
- Publication of clinical and scientific papers
- Audio and videocassette courses
- Teleclasses
- Distance education programs

References

1.	Hildebrandt RW. Chiropractic continuing education: A critical review. Am J Chiro Med 1989; 2(3):89-92.

2.	Rayles MD. Professional ethics. Wadsworth Publishing Co., Belmont, CA 1981; 75.

3.	Houle CO. Continuing learning in the professions. Jossey-Bass Publishers, San Francisco 1980; 76-123.

4.	Official Directory Federation of Chiropractic Licensing Boards. Greeley, CO, 1993.

5.	Council on Chiropractic Education. Standards for chiropractic institutions. West Des Moines, IA 1990; Council on Chiropractic Education.

6.	Davis I. Ethics: an analysis and a theory. J Chiro 1990; 27(4):20-23.

7.	Federation of Chiropractic Licensing Boards. Official Directory of the Federation of Chiropractic Licensing Boards. Kremmling, CO, Federation of Chiropractic Licensing Boards, 1989. Annual.

8.	Haldeman S, ed. Modern developments in the principles and practice of chiropractic: based on a conference sponsored by the International Chiropractors Association, Anaheim, CA, February 1979. New York, Appleton-Century-Crofts 1980; 390 pp.

9.	Haldeman S. Philosophy and the future of chiropractic. J Chiro 1990; 27(7):23-28.

10.	Kelner M, Hall O, Coulter I. Chiropractors: do they help? A study of their education and practice. Toronto, Fitzhenry & Whiteside 1980; 303 pp.

11.	Lawrence DJ. Research and responsibility. J Manipulative Physiol Ther 1984; 7(3):179-181.

12.	Mauer EL. Selected ethics and protocols in chiropractic. Gaithersburg, MD, Aspen Publishers 1991; 273 pp.

13.	Rosenthal SF. A sociology of chiropractic. Lewiston, NY, Edwin Mellen Press, 1986. 15 pp.

14.	Vear HJ, ed. Chiropractic standards of practice and quality of care. Gaithersburg, MD, Aspen Publishers, Incorrectly. 1991; 303 pp.

Contributors and Panel Members

Christopher Kent, D.C., F.C.C.I.
President, Council on Chiropractic Practice
Post-graduate Faculty
Life University, Marietta, Georgia
Ramsey, New Jersey

Named "Chiropractic Researcher of the Year" in 1994 by the World Chiropractic Alliance, and in 1991 by the International Chiropractors Association, Dr. Kent was one of only 16 chiropractors worldwide selected as a participant of the 1975 NINCDS workshop sponsored by the National Institutes of Health. He was a principal investigator in the Palmer College research department, where he served as assistant professor of diagnosis and x-ray. He has presented papers at scientific symposia including the PCCR CORE Conference, the Reviews of the Literature Conference, and the ICA Scientific Symposium on Spinal Biomechanics.

William Ralph Boone, Ph.D., D.C.
Vice President, Council on Chiropractic Practice
Editor, Journal of Vertebral Subluxation Research
Irvine, California

Formerly president of Southern California College of Chiropractic and director of research and computer resources at Sherman College of Chiropractic, Dr. Boone is now co-principal investigator for a research project at the University of California, Irvine. His work has appeared in numerous scientific journals and professional publications such as *Chiropractic Economics, Manipulative and Physiological Therapeutics, Chiropractic,* and *Technological Horizons in Education Journal.*

Terry A. Rondberg, D.C.
Secretary, Council on Chiropractic Practice
President, World Chiropractic Alliance
Chandler, Arizona

Founder and president of the World Chiropractic Alliance and publisher of *The Chiropractic Journal,* Dr. Rondberg was instrumental in the development of the Wyndham Guidelines. His work has appeared in numerous publications and he is known as a prolific writer and speaker. A 1974 graduate of Logan College of Chiropractic, Rondberg has authored several articles on chiropractic for both the profession and the public.

Harold G. McCoy, D.C.
Treasurer, Council on Chiropractic Practice
President, International Spinal Health Institute
Private Practice
Kirkland, Washington

This highly respected member of the World Chiropractic Alliance has sponsored all three previous Outcome Assessments and Diagnostics Symposiums and is program coordinator of this year's event His varied background includes strong experience in sports chiropractic, including seven years of service as a consultant to the University of Washington Intercollegiate Athletic Department. During the 1984 Olympics, he was chiropractor to the U.S. Olympic Boxing Team. In 1983, he was a member of the U.S. Olympic Medical Staff for the Pan American Games. Dr. McCoy, a Diplomate in Applied Chiropractic Sciences, has also served as chiropractor for the Boston Marathon and the Women's Marathon Olympic Trials.

Emmanuel T. Akporiaye, Ph.D.
Associate Professor of Microbiology and
 Immunology
Arizona Health Sciences Center
University of Arizona
Tucson, Arizona

An associate professor of microbiology and immunology at the Arizona Health Sciences Center in Tucson, Arizona, Dr. Akporiaye served as Commissioner of the Arizona Disease Control Research Commission and as a member of the National Institutes of Health Special Program Grant Review Committee. His work has been published in numerous medical and research journals.

Robert Blanks, Ph.D.
Professor, Department of Anatomy and
 Neurobiology
University of California, Irvine
Irvine, California

Before joining the Department of Anatomy and Neurobiology at the University of California, Irvine — where he is currently a professor — Dr. Blanks spent 10 years at the National Institutes of of Health and two years as visiting scientist at the Max Planck Institute for Brain Research in Frankfurt, Germany. His list of publishing credits include 56 manuscripts, 11 books or book chapters, and 82 abstracts.

Patrick Gentempo, D.C.
President, Chiropractic Leadership Alliance
Paterson, New Jersey

Dr. Gentempo is a member of the Board of Directors of the International Chiropractic Pediatric Association and the Council of New Jersey Chiropractors. He has served as a guest lecturer for numerous chiropractic colleges, including Palmer, Life, Logan and Parker. His work has been published in *International Review of Chiropractic, Chiropractic Research Journal, The Chiropractic Journal, Today's Chiropractic, The Journal of Chiropractic Research and Clinical Investigation,* and numerous other professional publications.

John J. Gerhardt, M.D.
Consultant in Physical Medicine and Rehabilitation
Shriners Hospital and Veterans Affairs Hospital
  Medical Center
Portland, Oregon

Tackling the topic, "Validating Clinical Outcomes by Objective and Comparable Range of Motion Measurements," Dr. Gerhardt completed his orthopedic residency in Vienna and was board certified in orthopedics in 1956. He is a member of the worker's compensation committee of the Oregon Medical Association and consultant to the American Medical School and the American Medical Association in preparation of the Guide to the Evaluation of Permanent Impairment 14th ed. He has published papers and books in orthopedic measurement and documentation and co-authored several books in orthopedic disease, examination, standardization of measurements and diagnostics in orthopedics and traumatology. He is a consultant in Physical Medicine and Rehabilitation at Shriners Hospital and Veterans Affairs Hospital Medical Center in Portland.

Veronica Gutierrez, D.C.
Member of the Washington State Quality
  Assurance Commission
Private Practice
Arlington, Washington

A graduate of Palmer College of Chiropractic, Dr. Gutierrez has long been active in managed health care issues with the United Chiropractors of Washington. Recently appointed a member of the Washington State Board of Chiropractic Examiners, she also chairs the Health Care Reform Committee for the World Chiropractic Alliance and is a contributing editor for *The Chiropractic Journal.* In addition, she chaired the Managed Health Care Committee and served on the Standards of Care committee for the Washington State Chiropractic Association.

Jonathan Hatch, Esquire
Member Washington State Bar Association
Member Snohomish County Bar Association
Lynnwood, Washington

Mr. Hatch received his Doctor of Jurisprudence degree from Willamette University College of Law in 1972. Following his admission to the practice of law in Washington state in 1972, he served four years as a Judge Advocate in the United States Marine Corps, including service as a Special Courts-Martial trial judge. He entered private law practice in 1977. In 1978 he co-founded a law firm in Lynnwood, Washington and served as its managing shareholder until 1996. He currently conducts his practice as a sole practitioner in Lynnwood, Washington. He is a member of the Washington State Bar Association and the Snohomish County Bar Association. Mr. Hatch's practice has included defense of professional negligence cases, personal injury, and professional licensing and discipline matters. He has been published in *The Chiropractic Journal,* and is a member of the Editorial Board of the *Journal of Vertebral Subluxation Research.* He serves as a member of the Board of Directors of the Council on Chiropractic Practice and of the International Spinal Health Institute.

Jay Holder, D.C., M.D., Ph.D.
President, American College of Addictionology
  and Compulsive Disorders
Private Practice
Miami Beach, Florida
Winner of the Albert Schweitzer prize in medicine and president/co-founder of the American College of Addictionology and Compulsive Disorders. Dr. Holder was awarded the Dag Hammerskjold Fellowship by the Academis Diplomatique de la Paix. He also holds appointment to the faculty, Pharmacology Department at the University of Miami. Holder is presently investigating the efficacy of chiropractic in addiction treatment and is developing the "Brain Reward Cascade," a model supporting the vertebral subluxation complex.

Carol James
Consumer Member
Bellevue, Washington
Serving as a consumer member of the board, James is actively involved in community service including volunteer work with the U.S. Olympic Committee, the University of Washington Hall of Fame, United Way, Senior Citizens, March of Dimes and numerous other organizations. Her professional background includes television and radio broadcast work.

Matthew McCoy, D.C.
Vice President, International Spinal Health Institute
Private Practice
Kirkland, Washington
A private practitioner from Florida, Dr. McCoy is a 1989 graduate of Life College. He has extensive post-graduate education, including training in Upper Cervical Specific Technique, Acquired Immuno-Deficiency Syndrome, Outcomes Assessment, and Vertebral Subluxation. He holds licenses in three states and is a certified Independent Medical Examiner.

Stephen F. Renner, D.C.
Member American Board of Forensic Examiners
Private Practice
Spokane, Washington
A 1976 graduate of Palmer College of Chiropractic, Dr. Renner is certified in surface EMG and videofluoroscopy. His post-graduate training includes the Council on Applied Chiropractic Science diplomate program, as well as study in applied spinal biomechanical engineering. A member of the American Board of Forensic Examiners and the American Academy of Pain Management, Renner has presented seminars for the Washington Defense Trial Lawyers and the Montana State Trial Lawyers Association Convention.

Steven Shochat, D.C.
Private Practice
Tucson, Arizona

A past member of the Board of Directors of the Arizona Association of Chiropractors, Dr. Shochat has been in private practice since 1981. He served as a member of the steering committee for the Wyndham Conference as well as the World Chiropractic Alliance panel on vertebral subluxation.

Technique Conference Participants

Applied Kinesiology
Richard Belli, D.C.
Shawnee Mission, KS

Applied Spinal
 Biomechanics Engineering
Donald W. Olson, D.C.
Auburn, WA

Atlas Orthogonality
Peter Garibaldi, D.C.
Phoenix, AZ

Association of Upper Cervical
 Chiropractic Organizations
Hal Crowe, D.C.
Brunswick, GA

Barge Technique
Fred Barge, D.C.
LaCrosse WI

Bio-energetic Synchronization
 Technique
M.T. Morter, Jr., D.C.
Rogers, AR

Blair Technique
George Banitch, D.C.
Montclair, NJ

Directional Non-Force Technique
Harlan Sparer, D.C.
Sedona, AZ

Freeman Chiropractic Seminars
Michael Freeman, D.C.
Salem, OR

Gonstead
Larry Troxell, D.C.
Parkview, IA

Kale Research and Technology
Frank Iulianelli, D.C.
Spartanburg, SC

Network Spinal Analysis
Donald Epstein, D.C.
Boulder, CO

Neuro Emotional Technique
Scott Walker, D.C.
Encinatas, CA

Neural Organizational Technique
Carl Ferreri, D.C.
Brooklyn, NY

Nimmo Recepter Tonus Technique
Sheila Laws, D.C.
Quincy, IL

National Upper Cervical
 Chiropractic Association
Albert Berti, D.C.
Burnaby, British Columbia, Canada

Orthospinology
Kirk Eriksen, D.C.
Dothan, AL

Pettibon Technique
Raymond Weigand, D.C.
Garland, TX

Pierce Stillwagon Technique
Glenn Stillwagon, D.C.
Monongahala, PA

Stressology
Lowell Ward, D.C.
Long Beach, CA

The Upledger Institute
Charles Kirkman, D.C.
Mesa, AZ

Thompson Technique
Beth Zogg, D.C.
Augusta, GA

Toftness Technique
David Toftness, D.C.
Amery, WI

Torque Release Technique
Jay Holder, D.C.
Miami Beach, FL

Total Body Modification
Francis Remedios, D.C.
Redding, CA

Vickery Method
Brice Vickery, D.C.
West Redding, CT

Leadership Conference Participants

Claudia Anrig, D.C.
Fresno, CA

J.J. Chatrouse, D.C.
San Rafael, CA

Gary Dunn, D.C.
Nashville, TN

Chuck Gibson, D.C.
Laguna Hills, CA

Ian Grassam, D.C.
Stuart, FL

Greg Jack
Mesa, AZ

Dennis Perman, D.C.
Huntington, NY

Dick Plummer, D.C.
Boiling Springs, SC

Garry Pomeroy
Pennsauken, NJ

David Singer, D.C.
Clearwater, FL

Greg Stanley
Phoenix, AZ

Peer Reviewers

Peter Amlinger, D.C.
Mississauga Ont, Canada

Jay Lepp, D.C.
Coquitlam BC, Canada

Elizabeth Anderson-Peacock, D.C.
Barrie Ont, Canada

Jean-Jacques Lob, D.C.
Villasanta, Italy

Mark Baerwaldt, D.C.
Milano, Italy

Ernest P. Miron, D.C.
Winnipeg MB, Canada

Albert Berti, D.C.
Burnaby BC, Canada

Brett Moore, D.C.
Oakville Ont, Canada

Richard R. Bray, D.C.
Windsor Ont, Canada

Jamie Neely, D.C.
London Ont, Canada

Johanna Carlo, D.C.
Toronto Ont, Canada

Rolf Osthus, D.C.
Levanger, Norway

Tony Croke, D.C.
Gisborne Vic, Australia

Ingjerd Osthus, D.C.
Levanger, Norway

Ari Diskin, D.C.
Fitzroy Vic, Australia

Mark Postles, D.C.
Budding QLD, Australia

Matthew Flanagan, D.C.
Neuwry County, Northern Ireland

Mark Preyser, D.C.
Kenilworth, South Africa

Peter Gyrst, D.C.
Odense, Denmark

Mike Pyfron, D.C.
Nassau, Bahamas

Karina Gyrst, D.C.
Odense, Denmark

Peter Robb, D.C.
Mittagona NSW, Australia

Henrik Gyrst, D.C.
Odense, Denmark

Christina Rodes, D.C.
Alderley QLD, Australia

Brad Harper, D.C.
Grand Cayman Island

Susan Shaw, D.C.
Barrie Ont, Canada

Cameron Harrison, D.C.
Edison AB, Canada

John E. K. Stevens, D.C.
Nassau, Bahamas

Ely Lazar, D.C.
Shenton Park WA, Australia

Lynn Stevens, D.C.
Nassau, Bahamas

Greg Stiles, D.C.
Edmonton, AB, Canada

Jim Stinear, D.C.
Auckland, New Zealand

Mike Storey, D.C.
Peterborough Ont, Canada

Robert Straub, D.C.
Janschwalde, Germany

Robin Taylor, D.C.
Takapuna Auckland, New Zealand

Sinclair Warner, D.C.
Southerwood East London, So. Africa

Rod Weiland, D.C.
Chatswood NSW, Australia

David Whitfield, D.C.
Port Elizabeth, South Africa

James Pizzadilli, D.C.
Anchorage, AK

Kirt Ericksen, D.C.
Dothan, AL

Willard Johnson, D.C.
Cullman, AL

Samuel Haley, D.C.
Little Rock, AR

Richard J. Aragon, D.C.
Tucson, AZ

David J. Brotman, D.C.
Mesa, AZ

Gregory Hertzberg, D.C.
Chandler, AZ

Bruce Homsey, D.C.
Glendale, AZ

Fred Schofield, D.C.
Glendale, AZ

Robert W. Adams, D.C.
Sonoma, CA

Joe Awender, II, D.C.
Redwood City, CA

Bart Bishop, D.C.
Whittier, CA

Erich Breitenmoser, D.C.
Temecula, CA

James R. Caballero, D.C.
Oxnard, CA

Frederick A. Carbone, D.C.
Santa Maria, CA

Jean-Jaques Chatrousse, D.C.
San Rafael, CA

David E. Cox, D.C.
Bluff, CA

Jason A. Deitch, D.C.
Oakland, CA

Dusan Djukich, D.C.
Dixon, CA

Lonney D. Edwards, D.C.
Fresno, CA

Chuck Gibson, D.C.
Laguna Hills, CA

Dean Kerr, D.C.
Chino, CA

Mark Kimes, D.C.
Salines, CA

Rayce Meyers, D.C.
San Mateo, CA

Brian Patrick Miller, D.C.
Crescenta, CA

David Shores, D.C.
Encinitas, CA

Scott Walker, D.C.
Encinatas, CA

Jerry L. Wood, D.C.
Citrus Heights, CA

Brian Zaleski, D.C.
Vacaville, CA

Donald Epstein, D.C.
Boulder, CO

Scott White, D.C.
Ft. Collins, CO

Donald Mears, D.C.
Enfield, CT

Alan Lichter, D.C.
Washington, DC

Terry Findley, D.C.
Dover, DE

Brian Burns, D.C.
Tampa, FL

Thomas C. D'Amico, D.C.
Davie, FL

Henry M. Rubinstein, D.C.
Miami, FL

Michael West Shreeve, D.C.
Tampa, FL

David Singer, D.C.
Clearwater, FL

Robert Braile, D.C.
Powder Springs, GA

Hal Crowe, D.C.
Brunswick, GA

Bruce Grundy, D.C.
Peachtree City, GA

D.D. Humber, D.C.
Marietta, GA

Richard A. Pistolese D.C.
Atlanta, GA

Rhody Edwards, D.C.
Kailua-Kona, HI

Nicholas Opie, Jr., DC
Kailua, HI

R. Douglas Baker, D.C.
Davenport, IA

Jeffrey Shay, D.C.
Muscatine, IA

Christopher I. Thornell, D.C.
Hiawatha, IA

Larry Troxell, D.C.
Parkview, IA

Norris Erickson, D.C.
Aurora, IL

David Ginsberg, D.C.
Geneva, IL

Peter Zid, D.C.
Chicago, IL

Wayne B. Ladd, D.C.
Bunker Hill, IN

Andrew Wymore, D.C.
Overland, KS

Dennis Heskett, D.C.
Murray, KY

Paul Johnston, D.C.
Shreveport, LA

Angela Gambale, D.C.
Swampscott, MA

Michael R. Girard, D.C.
Hudson, MA

Christopher Cianci, D.C.
Easton, MD

William Lawler, D.C.
Waterville, ME

Warren B. Atkinson, D.C.
Chelsea, MI

Karl R.O.S. Johnson, D.C.
Shelby Township, MI

David J. Klida, D.C.
East Pointe, MI

Michael J. Kudlas, D.C.
Kalamazoo, MI

Gary R. McLeon, D.C.
Three Rivers, MI

John R. Currier, D.C.
Burnsville, MN

Kevin M. Baum, D.C.
Ballwin, MO

George Goodman, D.C.
Chesterfield, MO

David L. Rozeboom, D.C.
St. Louis, MO

Roger Gregory, D.C.
Jackson, MS

Jim Brandau, D.C.
Livingston, MT

Spence J. Jahner, D.C.
Bozeman, MT

Donald Acton, D.C.
Asheville, NC

Robert McCarthy, D.C.
Greenville, NC

Curtis Ficenec, D.C.
Fargo, ND

David Kats, D.C.
Lincoln, NE

James P. Shearman, D.C.
Omaha, NE

Michael Clark, D.C.
Rochester, NH

Joshua J. Joaquin, D.C.
Rindge, NH

George Banitch, D.C.
Montclair, NJ

Susan K. Dorgai, D.C.
Glen Gardner, NJ

Jim Dubel, D.C.
Red Bank, NJ

Elliott Foster, D.C.
E. Rutherford, NJ

Glenn Gabai, D.C.
Pennington, NJ

Michael Manginelli, D.C.
Irvington, NJ

Keith J. O'Connell, D.C.
Waldwick, NJ

Darrell Atchley, D.C.
Lovington, NM

Phillip Goforth, D.C.
Socorro, NM

Herbert Reaver, D.C.
Pisgah, OH

Teresa Berry, D.C.
Las Vegas, NV

Laura Sparks, D.C.
Athens, OH

Darren R. Bell, D.C.
Derby, NY

Harold Culver, D.C.
Marlow, OK

Lisa K. Bloom, D.C.
Waterloo, NY

John Cafferty, D.C.
Gresham, OR

William V. Brennan, D.C.
Seaford, NY

Brian Stearns, D.C.
Salem, OR

Allan Cherkin, D.C.
Patchogue, NY

James Warner, D.C.
Keizer, OR

Joseph Clauss, D.C.
Plattsburg, NY

Gregg J. Fisher, D.C.
Montoursville, PA

Stephen R. Goldman, D.C.
Hicksville, NY

David T. Gruda, D.C.
Erie, PA

Robert Hoffman, D.C.
Oyster Bay, NY

Ernest Laubach, D.C.
Muncy, PA

John Incledon, D.C.
Fishkill, NY

Mark D. Losagio, D.C.
Bethleham, PA

David Kerschner, D.C.
E. Greenbush, NY

Wesley Mullen, Jr., D.C.
Mountaintop, PA

Dennis Perman, D.C.
Huntington, NY

Lee A. Newman, D.C.
Pittsburgh, PA

John Russo, D.C.
Oakdale, NY

Nick Spano, D.C.
Canton, PA

Jay H. Schwartz, D.C.
Pomere, NY

Jack K. Van Dervort, D.C.
Meadville, PA

Lawrence J. Suchoff, D.C.
New City, NY

James M. Wehner, D.C.
Pittsburgh, PA

Craig Longworth, D.C.
Akron, OH

Richard A. Barone, D.C.
Williamston, SC

Kenneth A. Curtis, D.C.
Rock Hill, SC

Bobby D. Findley, Jr., D.C.
Myrtle Beach, SC

Harvey Garcia, D.C.
Anderson, SC

Michael Kale, D.C.
Spartanburg, SC

David Koch, D.C.
Spartanburg, SC

Marvin Braun, D.C.
Gregory, SD

Max Reinecke, D.C.
Sioux Falls, SD

Joseph F. Amato, D.C.
Kingsport, TN

Richard J. Stephenson, D.C.
Bryan, TX

Michael Cerami, D.C.
Salt Lake City, UT

Michael P. Amato, D.C.
Staunton, VA

Pippa R. Chapman, D.C.
Pearisbours, VA

Michael Henderson, D.C.
Herndon, VA

Charles Masarsky, D.C.
Vienna, VA

Bradbury Robinson, D.C.
Norfolk, VA

Marion Weber, D.C.
Vienna, VA

Sean P. Mahoney, D.C.
Colchester, VT

John Babich, D.C.
Kent, WA

Jay M. Baker, D.C.
Federal Way, WA

John S. Blye, D.C.
Lynnwood, WA

Michael Clusserath, D.C.
Kent, WA

James O. Hagen, D.C.
Spokane, WA

James Milliron, D.C.
Yakima, WA

Donald W. Olson, D.C.
Auburn, WA

Fred Barge, D.C.
Lacrosse, WI

James R. Bowman, D.C.
Plover, WI

Dale Kenney, D.C.
Algona, WI

J.G. Moellendorf, D.C.
Sturgeon Bay, WI

Mark A. Pederson, D.C.
Hudson, WI

Joseph J. Teff, D.C.
Middleton, WI

David Toftness, D.C.
Amery, WI

Gordon Toftness, D.C.
Amery, WI

L

Leg length inequality 4
Low velocity thrust 74

M

Magnetic resonance imaging (MRI) 41
Manually assisted mechanical thrust 74
Mental health outcomes 3, 5
Modes of adjustive care 73, 74
Moiré contourography 20
Motion palpation 4
Muscle testing
    computerized 23
    manual 23

N

Neurological examination 5

O

Orthopedic examination 5
Outcomes assessment 65

P

Pain 3, 21
Palpation 4
Patient safety 95-97
Pediatric chiropractic 87-90
Physical examination 59
Plumb line 4, 19
Postural analysis 19
Practice objective 95
Professional development 101

Q

Quality of Life 24, 65
Questionnaires 24, 65

R

Radiographic imaging 39, 40
Radioisotope scanning 43
Range of motion 20
Rating system xi
Reassessment 65
Recoil 74
Re-examination 65
Referral 96

Retrospective review 59

S

Safety, patient 95-97
Satisfaction, patient 24, 65
Scales, bilateral and four-quadrant 20
Skin temperature instrumentation 22
Somatosensory evoked potentials
  (SSEP) 22
Spinography —
  see radiographic imaging
Stroke 96, 97
Substance abuse 3, 5
Surface electromyography (SEMG) 23

T

Terms of acceptance 95
Thermocouple instruments 22
Thermography 22
Thrust 73, 74
Toggle 74
Toggle recoil 75
Tone 74
Torque 75

U

Ultrasonography 42

V

Videofluoroscopy 40, 41

W

Weight scales 20

X

X-ray — see radiographic imaging